Embracing Social Norms: The Psychology of Human Interaction

Laurel D. Malvern

Copyright and Legal Disclaimer

Preface

Welcome to "Embracing Social Norms: The Psychology of Human Interaction." In this book, we embark on a captivating journey through the intricate landscape of social psychology, exploring how norms, behaviors, and relationships shape our everyday lives.

Social psychology is a discipline that delves into the dynamics of human behavior within social contexts. It seeks to unravel the complexities of why we think, feel, and act the way we do when interacting with others. Through this exploration, we gain profound insights into ourselves and the world around us.

I have crafted this book to serve as a comprehensive guide for students, professionals, and curious minds alike. Each chapter is meticulously designed to build upon the foundations of social psychology, offering a blend of theoretical frameworks, empirical research, and practical applications.

Our journey begins with an exploration of the fundamental definitions and scope of social psychology, setting the stage for deeper insights into the importance of understanding human behavior through a social lens. From the roles of social interactions in daily life to the complexities of mental health and social support systems, we uncover the various facets that influence our social experiences.

Throughout these pages, we delve into the nature of relationships, the psychology of emotions, and the profound impact of communication on interpersonal dynamics. We navigate through the nuances of self-esteem, group dynamics, and the persuasive power of social influence, all while examining how social norms dictate our behaviors and identities.

In our quest to understand human interaction, we also confront challenging topics such as prejudice, stereotypes, and the formation of social identities. We explore the role of empathy in fostering meaningful connections and examine the cognitive processes that shape our perceptions of others.

This book is not merely an academic exploration but a journey of personal reflection and growth. It challenges us to think critically about the social norms that govern our lives and encourages us to consider how we can shape and redefine these norms to foster inclusivity and understanding.

As we reach the conclusion, we reflect on the interconnectedness of the concepts explored throughout this book. We contemplate the implications of social psychology for personal development, professional practice, and future research endeavors.

I invite you to embark on this journey with an open mind and a curiosity for understanding the complexities of human social behavior. May this book serve as a guidepost in your quest to navigate the intricate tapestry of human interaction and connection.

With warm regards,

Laurel D. Malvern

Introduction: The Essence of Social Psychology

Welcome to "Embracing Social Norms: The Psychology of Human Interaction." In this introduction, we embark on a profound exploration of social psychology — a discipline that illuminates the complex interplay between individuals and their social environments.

Social psychology delves into how our thoughts, feelings, and behaviors are shaped by the presence of others. It seeks to unravel the intricate dynamics of human interaction, shedding light on why we behave differently in social settings, how group dynamics influence decision-making, and the psychological mechanisms behind interpersonal relationships.

At its core, social psychology provides a lens through which we can understand the fundamental aspects of human nature within social contexts. We examine the role of social norms—unwritten rules that guide behavior—in shaping our attitudes and actions. These norms not only dictate what is considered acceptable in society but also influence our identities and sense of belonging.

Throughout this book, we will explore a diverse range of topics essential to social psychology. We will delve into the psychology of communication, examining how verbal and nonverbal cues impact our interactions and relationships. We will explore the dynamics of emotions and their regulation, considering how emotional intelligence contributes to social success and well-being.

Furthermore, we will investigate the psychological underpinnings of identity formation, examining how individuals develop a sense of self within the context of their social groups and cultures. Topics such as self-esteem, social cognition, and the perception of others will provide insights into how our thoughts about ourselves and others shape our social behaviors.

As we navigate through these chapters, we will also confront challenging issues such as prejudice, stereotyping, and the dynamics of social influence. We will discuss strategies for promoting empathy, challenging social norms, and fostering inclusive communities.

Ultimately, this book aims to not only deepen your understanding of social psychology but also to inspire reflection and critical thinking about the social world around you. Whether you are a student embarking on your academic journey, a professional seeking insights into human behavior, or simply a curious reader fascinated by the complexities of social interaction, this exploration promises to offer both theoretical insights and practical applications.

Join me as we embark on this intellectual journey through social psychology, where each chapter offers new perspectives and discoveries that will enhance your appreciation of the rich tapestry of human social behavior.

Welcome to the world of "Embracing Social Norms: The Psychology of Human Interaction."

Warm regards,

Laurel D. Malvern

Chapter 1: Introduction to Social Psychology

Social psychology is the scientific study of how individuals' thoughts, feelings, and behaviors are influenced by the actual, imagined, or implied presence of others. It seeks to understand the dynamics of human interaction within various social contexts, ranging from everyday interactions to complex group dynamics and societal influences.

Definition: Social psychology emerged as a distinct field in the early 20th century, influenced by both psychology and sociology. Unlike sociology, which focuses on larger societal structures and institutions, social psychology emphasizes the individual's psychological processes in social situations.

Evolution: The field has evolved significantly since its inception, adapting to incorporate advances in psychology, neuroscience, and other disciplines. Early theories focused on individual behaviors in social situations, while contemporary social psychology integrates cognitive, behavioral, and neuroscientific approaches to study social phenomena.

Interdisciplinary Nature: Social psychology intersects with other disciplines such as sociology, anthropology, neuroscience, and economics. This interdisciplinary approach allows researchers to explore complex social issues from multiple perspectives, enriching our understanding of human behavior.

Theoretical Frameworks
Social Cognition: This theoretical framework examines how individuals perceive, interpret, and remember information about themselves and others in social contexts. It explores cognitive processes such as attention, memory, and judgment that influence social perception and decision-making.

Social Influence: This framework focuses on how the presence and actions of others (real, imagined, or implied) shape individual behavior, attitudes, and beliefs. It encompasses concepts like conformity, compliance, and obedience, as well as the study of persuasion and group dynamics.

Social Identity Theory: Developed by Tajfel and Turner, this theory explores how individuals derive their sense of identity from group memberships and how group membership influences behavior and attitudes. It addresses issues of prejudice, intergroup relations, and collective identity.

Methodological Approaches
Experiments: Experimental research designs allow researchers to manipulate variables and establish cause-and-effect relationships. Social psychologists use experiments to study how changes in social conditions (e.g., presence of others, social norms) affect behavior.

Surveys: Surveys and questionnaires are commonly used to collect self-reported data on attitudes, beliefs, and behaviors. They provide insights into how individuals perceive social situations and their responses to social stimuli.

Observational Studies: Observational research involves systematically recording behaviors in naturalistic settings without intervention. This method allows researchers to study behavior in real-world contexts and observe natural social interactions.

Qualitative Approaches: Qualitative methods such as interviews and focus groups explore the richness and depth of social experiences, attitudes, and beliefs. They provide nuanced insights into individuals' subjective experiences and perceptions.

Scope and Applications
Micro-level Interactions: Social psychology examines individual behaviors in everyday social interactions, such as impression formation, interpersonal attraction, and social perception. It explores how social norms and situational factors influence behavior on a personal level.

Macro-level Influences: At a macro level, social psychology investigates societal influences on behavior and attitudes, including cultural norms, social institutions, and political ideologies. It explores how broader social forces shape collective behavior and societal change.

Applications: Social psychology has practical applications in various domains, including health psychology (e.g., promoting healthy behaviors), organizational psychology (e.g., improving workplace dynamics), and environmental psychology (e.g., encouraging pro-environmental behaviors). It informs interventions aimed at addressing social issues and improving well-being.

Ethical Considerations
Informed Consent: Researchers must obtain voluntary and informed consent from participants, explaining the study's purpose, procedures, risks, and benefits before participation.

Confidentiality: Protecting participants' confidentiality ensures that their personal information remains secure and anonymous, minimizing potential harm or stigma.

Minimizing Harm: Researchers are obligated to minimize potential physical, psychological, or social harm to participants during the study.

Ethical Guidelines: Social psychologists adhere to ethical guidelines set by professional organizations (e.g., American Psychological Association) to ensure responsible conduct and integrity in research practices.

Conclusion

Chapter 1 lays the foundation for understanding the breadth and depth of social psychology. It introduces key concepts, theoretical frameworks, methodological approaches, and ethical considerations that guide the study of human behavior in social contexts. By exploring these elements, social psychology offers valuable insights into the complexities of interpersonal relationships, group dynamics, and societal influences.

This chapter sets the stage for deeper explorations in subsequent chapters, where we will examine specific topics such as social interactions, mental health, relationships, communication, and more. Join us as we continue to unravel the intricate tapestry of human social behavior in "Embracing Social Norms: The Psychology of Human Interaction."

Chapter 2: Connection Between Social Environments and Mental Health

Social Interactions: Social psychology emphasizes the significant impact of social interactions on individuals' psychological well-being. Positive social interactions, such as receiving support from friends or family, can enhance mood, reduce stress, and contribute to overall mental health. Conversely, negative interactions or social isolation may increase feelings of loneliness, anxiety, and depression.

Support Systems: Social support refers to the resources (emotional, instrumental, informational) provided by others during times of need or stress. Research in social psychology highlights the protective role of social support in buffering against the adverse effects of life stressors. For example, having supportive relationships can mitigate the impact of traumatic events or chronic stress on mental health.

Social Norms and Mental Health: Social norms—implicit or explicit rules governing acceptable behaviors within a group—also play a crucial role in mental health. Adherence to societal norms can influence individuals' self-perception and social identity, affecting their emotional well-being. Deviation from social norms may lead to social stigma or ostracism, which can negatively impact mental health outcomes.

Social Support Systems
Types of Social Support:

Emotional Support: Involves expressions of empathy, love, trust, and care from others. Emotional support helps individuals cope with emotional distress and promotes feelings of security and belonging.

Instrumental Support: Practical assistance or tangible resources provided by others, such as financial aid, transportation, or childcare. Instrumental support helps individuals manage daily tasks and navigate challenging situations.

Informational Support: Guidance, advice, or information provided by others to help individuals make informed decisions or solve problems. Informational support enhances individuals' ability to cope with stressors and make effective choices.

Effects of Social Support:

Health Benefits: Research indicates that strong social support networks are associated with better physical health outcomes, such as lower incidence of chronic diseases and faster recovery from illnesses.

Psychological Resilience: Social support enhances psychological resilience by fostering adaptive coping strategies and reducing the negative impact of stressors on mental health.

Longevity: Studies suggest that individuals with robust social connections tend to live longer than those who are socially isolated, highlighting the protective effects of social support on overall well-being.

The Impact of Stigma on Mental Health

Definition of Stigma: Stigma refers to negative attitudes, beliefs, and stereotypes associated with certain attributes or identities. In the context of mental health, stigma can lead to discrimination, social exclusion, and barriers to accessing mental health services.

Internalized Stigma: Individuals experiencing mental health challenges may internalize societal stigma, leading to feelings of shame, self-blame, and low self-esteem. Internalized stigma can hinder help-seeking behaviors and exacerbate psychological distress.

Barriers to Treatment: Stigma surrounding mental illness often creates barriers to seeking and receiving adequate treatment. Fear of being labeled, concerns about confidentiality, and perceived discrimination from healthcare providers may deter individuals from seeking professional help.

Addressing Stigma: Social psychology explores strategies to combat stigma and promote mental health awareness. These include education campaigns, advocacy for policy change, and fostering supportive environments that encourage open dialogue about mental health issues.

Practical Applications
Interventions: Social psychologists develop and evaluate interventions aimed at enhancing social support networks and reducing stigma associated with mental health. These interventions may involve community-based programs, psychoeducational workshops, and online support groups to promote resilience and well-being.

Policy Implications: Understanding the impact of social environments on mental health has significant policy implications. Policymakers can implement initiatives to strengthen social support systems, improve access to mental health services, and promote inclusive communities that respect and support individuals' mental health needs.

Conclusion

Chapter 2 underscores the critical role of social psychology in elucidating the complex interplay between social environments and mental health. By exploring the connections between social interactions, support systems, and stigma, social psychology provides valuable insights into promoting resilience, well-being, and inclusive communities.

Join us as we continue to unravel the dynamics of human behavior within social contexts in "Embracing Social Norms: The Psychology of Human Interaction."

Chapter 3: Interactions – The Fabric of Social Life

1. The Role of Social Interactions in Daily Life
Significance: Social interactions are fundamental to human existence and play a crucial role in shaping individuals' thoughts, emotions, and behaviors. From simple greetings to deep conversations, social interactions provide opportunities for connection, learning, and mutual support.

Functions:

Socialization: Interactions facilitate the transmission of cultural norms, values, and behaviors from one generation to the next. Through interactions with family, peers, and society, individuals learn appropriate conduct and societal expectations.

Communication: Social interactions involve verbal and nonverbal exchanges that convey information, emotions, and intentions. Effective communication skills are essential for building relationships and resolving conflicts.

Relationship Building: Interactions foster the development and maintenance of relationships. Whether familial, romantic, or platonic, interpersonal interactions strengthen social bonds and contribute to emotional well-being.

Impact: Positive social interactions contribute to happiness, fulfillment, and psychological resilience. Conversely, lack of social interaction or negative interactions can lead to feelings of loneliness, isolation, and distress.

2. Types of Social Interactions

Casual Interactions: Brief encounters characterized by low intimacy and spontaneity, such as exchanging greetings with strangers or making small talk with acquaintances.

Close Relationships: Intimate interactions involving deep emotional bonds and high levels of trust and disclosure. Examples include interactions with close friends, romantic partners, or family members.

Group Dynamics: Interactions within larger social groups or communities, involving coordination, cooperation, and conflict resolution. Group dynamics influence decision-making, conformity, and collective behaviors.

Professional Interactions: Interactions in work or organizational settings, focusing on task completion, teamwork, and professional relationships. Effective communication and collaboration are crucial for workplace success.

Community Interactions: Interactions within local communities or social networks, contributing to civic engagement, social support, and community development.

Virtual Interactions: Increasingly relevant in the digital age, interactions mediated through online platforms or social media. Virtual interactions impact social relationships, communication patterns, and identity formation.

3. Theories and Models Explaining Interactions

Social Exchange Theory: Posits that individuals engage in interactions based on a cost-benefit analysis, seeking to maximize rewards (e.g., companionship, support) while minimizing costs (e.g., time, effort).

Social Constructionism: Emphasizes the role of language and shared meanings in shaping social interactions and identities. Reality is socially constructed through mutual agreement and negotiation.

Symbolic Interactionism: Focuses on how symbols (e.g., gestures, words) and shared meanings influence social interactions. Individuals interpret symbols and adjust their behaviors based on perceived meanings and social norms.

Transactional Model of Communication: Describes communication as a dynamic process involving encoding, transmission, decoding, and feedback. Effective communication requires mutual understanding and clarity of message delivery.

Practical Applications
Enhancing Social Skills: Social psychology interventions aim to improve interpersonal skills, such as active listening, empathy, and conflict resolution, to enhance the quality of social interactions.

Cultural Competence: Understanding cultural differences in communication styles and social norms promotes effective interactions across diverse communities and enhances cross-cultural understanding.

Group Dynamics Interventions: Techniques for fostering cooperation, leadership development, and conflict resolution within groups to optimize collective performance and cohesion.

Conclusion

Chapter 3 underscores the foundational role of social interactions in shaping human behavior, relationships, and societal dynamics. By exploring the functions, types, and theoretical underpinnings of social interactions, social psychology provides valuable insights into fostering meaningful connections and understanding interpersonal dynamics.

Join us as we continue to unravel the complexities of human social behavior in "Embracing Social Norms: The Psychology of Human Interaction."

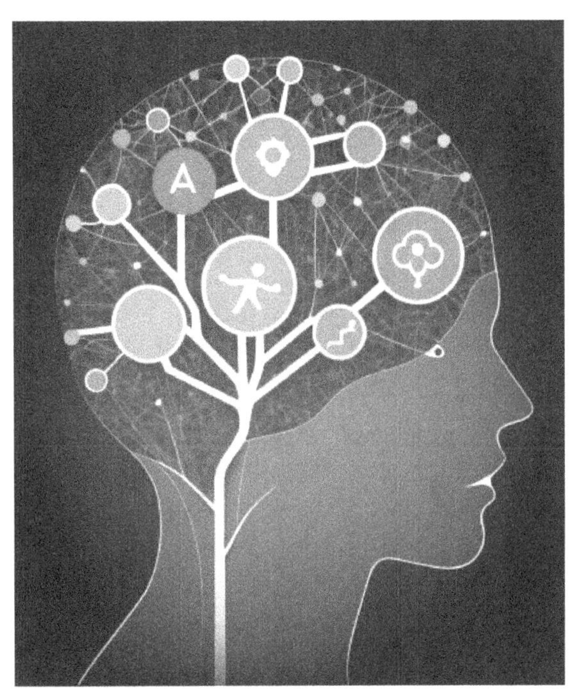

Chapter 4: The Role of Social Interactions in Daily Life

1. Functions of Social Interactions
Socialization:

Definition: Socialization refers to the process through which individuals acquire the knowledge, skills, values, and norms necessary to participate effectively in society.
Importance: From infancy to adulthood, social interactions with family members, peers, educators, and community members shape individuals' identities and social roles. Through socialization, individuals learn appropriate behaviors, language, and cultural practices.
Examples: Children learn societal norms through parental guidance, peer interactions teach social skills and cooperation, and community interactions reinforce cultural values.
Communication:

Verbal Communication: Involves the exchange of information, ideas, and emotions through spoken or written words. Effective verbal communication promotes understanding and fosters relationships.
Nonverbal Communication: Includes gestures, facial expressions, body language, and eye contact. Nonverbal cues enhance communication by conveying emotions, attitudes, and intentions.
Significance: Both verbal and nonverbal communication are essential for building rapport, resolving conflicts, and expressing empathy in interpersonal interactions.
Emotional Support:

Definition: Emotional support involves providing empathy, encouragement, and comfort to others during times of emotional distress or celebration.
Benefits: Receiving emotional support from friends, family, or community members enhances psychological well-being, reduces stress, and promotes resilience.
Role in Relationships: Close relationships characterized by emotional support foster trust, intimacy, and mutual dependency, contributing to overall life satisfaction and happiness.
2. Impact on Psychological Well-being
Happiness and Fulfillment:

Positive Interactions: Meaningful connections with others through social interactions contribute to feelings of happiness, fulfillment, and belonging.
Social Bonds: Close relationships provide emotional support, companionship, and shared experiences that enhance life satisfaction.
Research Findings: Studies consistently show that individuals with strong social ties report higher levels of happiness and overall well-being compared to those who are socially isolated.
Stress Reduction:

Buffering Effect: Supportive social networks serve as buffers against stress by providing emotional reassurance, practical assistance, and opportunities for distraction.
Health Benefits: Reduced stress levels associated with strong social support contribute to improved physical health outcomes, including lower blood pressure and better immune function.
Coping Mechanism: During challenging times, individuals rely on social interactions to cope with adversity and maintain psychological resilience.
Loneliness and Isolation:

Risk Factors: Lack of meaningful social interactions, social rejection, or perceived social isolation can lead to feelings of loneliness and emotional distress.

Health Consequences: Chronic loneliness is associated with increased risks of depression, anxiety, cardiovascular disease, and premature mortality.

Interventions: Addressing social isolation through community engagement, peer support programs, and mental health interventions promotes social connectedness and improves well-being.

3. Types of Social Interactions

Casual Interactions:

Examples: Brief exchanges with acquaintances, neighbors, or service providers (e.g., saying hello, small talk).

Functions: Foster a sense of community, maintain social norms, and provide opportunities for networking and relationship building.

Impact: Although low in intimacy, casual interactions contribute to social cohesion and community connectedness.

Close Relationships:

Characteristics: Intimate interactions characterized by trust, emotional closeness, and mutual support.

Types: Includes relationships with family members, close friends, romantic partners, and confidants.

Benefits: Close relationships fulfill emotional needs, provide social validation, and offer instrumental support during times of need.

Professional Interactions:

Workplace Context: Interactions with colleagues, supervisors, clients, and stakeholders in organizational settings.

Objectives: Facilitate task completion, collaboration on projects, and professional networking.

Skills: Effective communication, teamwork, and conflict resolution skills are crucial for building productive work relationships.

Practical Implications

Enhancing Social Skills:

Training Programs: Social psychology interventions focus on improving interpersonal skills such as active listening, empathy, assertiveness, and negotiation.

Application: Enhancing social skills promotes effective communication, builds rapport, and fosters positive interactions in personal and professional settings.

Promoting Social Support Networks:

Community Initiatives: Programs that encourage community involvement, peer support groups, and volunteer opportunities strengthen social ties and combat social isolation.

Health Benefits: Building and maintaining supportive relationships enhance mental health, emotional resilience, and overall quality of life.

Addressing Social Isolation:

Intervention Strategies: Outreach programs, mental health services, and social activities designed to reduce loneliness and promote social inclusion.

Community Engagement: Creating opportunities for social participation and fostering a sense of belonging in marginalized or isolated populations.

Conclusion

Chapter 4 underscores the pivotal role of social interactions in shaping individuals' daily lives, emotional well-being, and societal cohesion. By understanding the functions, impacts, and types of social interactions, individuals can cultivate meaningful relationships, mitigate loneliness, and contribute to a supportive and interconnected community.

Continue exploring the dynamics of human social behavior with us in "Embracing Social Norms: The Psychology of Human Interaction."

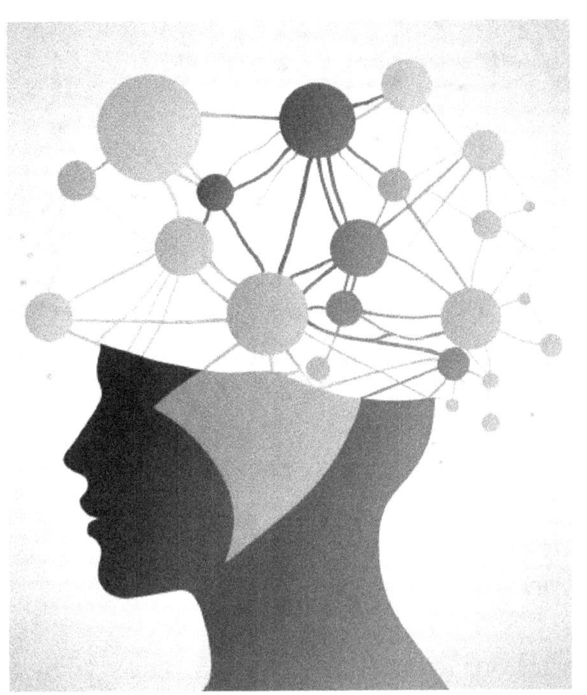

Chapter 5: Types of Social Interactions

Understanding the various types of social interactions is essential for grasping how individuals engage with others in different contexts. This chapter explores the nuances, roles, characteristics, and impacts of different types of social interactions on human behavior and relationships.

1. Casual Interactions
Definition and Characteristics:

Casual interactions are spontaneous, brief exchanges between individuals who may have minimal or no prior relationship. These interactions are typically informal and occur in everyday settings.
Examples: Casual interactions can include greetings with neighbors, small talk with colleagues in the workplace kitchen, or interactions with service providers such as cashiers or bus drivers.
Purpose: Despite their brevity, casual interactions play crucial roles in social dynamics. They help maintain social norms, establish a sense of community, and provide opportunities for networking.
Function: Casual interactions often serve as social lubricants, easing social tension and promoting a sense of belonging within a community or group.
2. Close Relationships
Definition and Characteristics:

Close relationships are characterized by strong emotional bonds, trust, and intimacy between individuals. These relationships involve deep personal connections and a high level of mutual support.

Types: Close relationships encompass familial bonds (e.g., with parents, siblings), romantic relationships (e.g., with partners or spouses), and close friendships.

Functions: Close relationships fulfill fundamental psychological needs for companionship, emotional validation, and social support.

Impact: Research consistently shows that individuals with supportive close relationships experience better mental health outcomes, higher life satisfaction, and increased resilience to stress.

3. Professional Interactions

Definition and Characteristics:

Professional interactions occur within formal settings such as workplaces, educational institutions, or professional networks. These interactions are goal-oriented and focus on achieving specific objectives.

Participants: Involve interactions between colleagues, supervisors, clients, customers, or stakeholders within organizational contexts.

Objectives: Professional interactions facilitate collaboration, decision-making processes, task completion, and maintaining professional relationships.

Skills: Effective communication, teamwork, negotiation, and conflict resolution skills are essential for navigating professional interactions successfully.

Impact: Strong professional relationships contribute to career advancement, job satisfaction, and organizational success.

4. Group Interactions

Definition and Characteristics:

Group interactions involve multiple individuals who come together based on shared goals, interests, or affiliations. Groups vary in size, structure, and purpose.

Functions: Group interactions serve various purposes such as social support, collective decision-making, problem-solving, and fostering a sense of belonging.

Examples: Groups can range from formal committees or project teams within organizations to informal social groups like clubs, sports teams, or community organizations.

Dynamics: Understanding group dynamics, roles, and norms is crucial for effective communication, collaboration, and cohesion within group settings.

Practical Implications

Enhancing Social Competence: Recognizing the diversity and dynamics of social interactions enables individuals to develop and refine their social skills. This includes skills such as empathy, active listening, assertiveness, adaptability, and conflict resolution.

Building Relationships: Understanding the nuances of different types of social interactions helps individuals cultivate and maintain meaningful relationships, whether personal or professional.

Promoting Inclusivity: Acknowledging the importance of diverse social interactions contributes to creating inclusive environments that value interpersonal connections and mutual respect.

Improving Well-being: Positive social interactions are linked to better psychological health, reduced stress levels, and increased overall well-being.

Conclusion

Chapter 5 underscores the significance of understanding the types of social interactions in navigating interpersonal relationships, professional environments, and community settings. By exploring the characteristics, functions, and impacts of casual interactions, close relationships, professional interactions, and group dynamics, individuals can enhance their social competence and contribute positively to social dynamics in various contexts.

Continue exploring the complexities of human social behavior in "Embracing Social Norms: The Psychology of Human Interaction."

Chapter 6: Theories and Models Explaining Interactions

Understanding human interactions requires delving into foundational theories and models that provide frameworks for comprehending how individuals connect, communicate, and behave in social settings. This chapter explores key theories and models, their principles, applications, and implications for understanding the dynamics of social interactions.

1. Social Exchange Theory
Definition and Principles:

Social Exchange Theory posits that individuals engage in interactions based on a rational assessment of costs and benefits. It suggests that people seek to maximize rewards (such as approval, support, resources) and minimize costs (such as time, effort, discomfort) in their social relationships.
Key Concepts:
Reciprocity: The exchange of resources or favors between individuals, where giving and receiving are balanced.

Equity: Fairness in the distribution of rewards and costs among participants.

Satisfaction: The subjective evaluation of whether outcomes meet expectations and fulfill needs.

Applications:

In interpersonal relationships, Social Exchange Theory explains how individuals negotiate intimacy, trust, and support.

In organizational behavior, it elucidates dynamics of reciprocity in teamwork, negotiations, and professional networks.

2. Symbolic Interactionism

Definition and Principles:

Symbolic Interactionism emphasizes the role of symbols and meanings in shaping social interactions. It posits that individuals create shared meanings through communication and interpretation of symbols (such as language, gestures, roles).

Key Concepts:

Symbols: Words, gestures, objects, or behaviors that carry shared meanings within a social group.

Meanings: Symbolic interpretations that guide behavior and influence social reality.

Identity and Self: Development of self-concept and identity through social interactions and symbolic communication.

Applications:

In sociology, Symbolic Interactionism explains how roles, identities, and social norms are constructed and negotiated.

In communication studies, it examines nonverbal cues, language use, and cultural symbols in interpersonal interactions.

3. Social Learning Theory

Definition and Principles:

Social Learning Theory proposes that individuals learn behaviors through observation, imitation, and reinforcement. It emphasizes the role of modeling and vicarious learning in acquiring social skills and behaviors.

Key Concepts:

Modeling: Observing and imitating behaviors exhibited by others, including peers, parents, and media figures.

Reinforcement: Rewards or punishments that reinforce or deter behaviors, influencing their repetition.

Vicarious Learning: Learning from the experiences and outcomes of others without direct personal experience.

Applications:

In education, Social Learning Theory informs teaching methods that emphasize modeling, peer learning, and positive reinforcement.

In behavioral psychology, it guides interventions for behavior modification, social skills training, and reducing aggression through observational learning.

4. Expectancy Violation Theory

Definition and Principles:

Expectancy Violation Theory explores how deviations from social norms and expectations influence perceptions and interactions. It examines the impact of unexpected behaviors on relational outcomes.

Key Concepts:

Personal Space: Cultural and individual expectations regarding physical proximity and spatial boundaries.

Communication Norms: Socially accepted rules and expectations governing verbal and nonverbal communication.

Socio-Cultural Context: Cultural, situational, and relational factors that shape expectations and responses to behavior.

Applications:

In interpersonal communication, Expectancy Violation Theory explains how violations of personal space or communication norms affect relational closeness or discomfort.

In cross-cultural studies, it helps understand how cultural differences in norms influence perceptions of behavior and interpersonal relationships.

Practical Implications

Enhancing Social Competence: Understanding these theories helps individuals develop effective social skills, including empathy, communication, negotiation, and conflict resolution.

Informing Interventions: Insights from these theories inform interventions aimed at improving interpersonal relationships, enhancing teamwork, and promoting positive social behaviors.

Advancing Research: Continued exploration and application of these theories contribute to advancing knowledge in social psychology, communication studies, and related fields, guiding future research and practical applications.

Conclusion

Chapter 6 provides a comprehensive exploration of key theories and models that explain human interactions in social contexts. By examining Social Exchange Theory, Symbolic Interactionism, Social Learning Theory, and Expectancy Violation Theory, individuals gain deeper insights into the dynamics of social behaviors, relational dynamics, and cultural influences. These theories not only enrich our understanding of human interaction but also offer practical implications for enhancing social relationships and promoting positive social change.

Continue exploring the complexities of human social behavior in "Embracing Social Norms: The Psychology of Human Interaction."

Chapter 7: The Impact of Stigma on Mental Health

Stigma surrounding mental health remains a significant barrier that affects individuals, communities, and societal attitudes toward mental illness. This chapter explores the pervasive effects of stigma on mental health outcomes, examining its origins, manifestations, and implications for individuals and society.

1. Understanding Stigma
Definition and Origins:

Stigma refers to negative attitudes, beliefs, and stereotypes that label individuals as different, flawed, or socially undesirable due to their mental health condition.
Origins: Stigma arises from societal prejudices, cultural norms, media portrayals, and historical perspectives that perpetuate misconceptions and discrimination against people with mental illness.
2. Forms of Stigma

Public Stigma:

Public Stigma involves widespread negative attitudes and beliefs held by the general population toward individuals with mental health disorders.
Manifestations: This stigma can lead to social exclusion, avoidance, labeling, and discrimination in employment, housing, and healthcare settings.
Self-Stigma:

Self-Stigma occurs when individuals internalize negative stereotypes and beliefs about mental illness, leading to diminished self-esteem, shame, and reluctance to seek help.
Impact: Self-stigma can undermine recovery efforts, reduce treatment adherence, and perpetuate feelings of isolation and hopelessness.
3. Consequences of Stigma
Barriers to Treatment:

Access and Utilization: Stigma creates barriers to accessing mental health services, leading to delayed treatment and underutilization of available resources.
Quality of Care: Individuals facing stigma may receive inadequate or discriminatory treatment from healthcare providers, impacting their overall health outcomes.
Social and Economic Impact:

Employment and Education: Stigma can affect employment opportunities, career advancement, and academic achievement due to discrimination and bias.
Family and Relationships: Stigma may strain family relationships and friendships, leading to social withdrawal and isolation.
4. Addressing Stigma
Education and Awareness:

Public Campaigns: Promoting awareness, challenging stereotypes, and fostering empathy through education and advocacy efforts.
Media Representation: Responsible media portrayal of mental health issues to reduce sensationalism and promote accurate understanding.
Policy and Legislation:

Legal Protections: Enacting anti-discrimination laws and policies that protect the rights of individuals with mental illness in employment, healthcare, and public accommodations.
Community Support: Building supportive communities that prioritize mental health awareness, acceptance, and inclusion.
Practical Implications
Promoting Resilience: Empowering individuals to challenge stigma, advocate for their rights, and seek support from peers and professionals.
Enhancing Treatment Outcomes: Integrating stigma-reduction strategies into mental health interventions to improve treatment adherence and recovery rates.
Advocacy and Social Change: Collaborating with stakeholders to promote systemic changes in attitudes, policies, and practices that perpetuate stigma.

Stigma surrounding mental health is a pervasive societal issue that profoundly affects individuals, communities, and healthcare systems. This chapter delves into the various facets of stigma, including its origins, forms, consequences, and strategies for addressing its impact on mental health.

1. Understanding Stigma
Definition and Origins:

Stigma refers to negative attitudes, beliefs, and stereotypes that lead to discrimination and social exclusion of individuals with mental health disorders. These attitudes are often rooted in societal prejudices, cultural norms, and historical misconceptions about mental illness.
Origins:

Stigma has historical roots dating back centuries, influenced by cultural beliefs, religious doctrines, and early medical theories that viewed mental illness as a sign of moral weakness or spiritual affliction rather than a medical condition requiring treatment.
2. Forms of Stigma
Public Stigma:

Public Stigma refers to the widespread negative attitudes and beliefs held by the general population toward individuals with mental illness. This type of stigma manifests in various ways, including fear, avoidance, labeling, and discriminatory behavior in social, educational, and employment settings.
Self-Stigma:

Self-Stigma occurs when individuals internalize societal stereotypes and negative beliefs about mental illness, leading to diminished self-esteem, shame, and reluctance to seek help. Self-stigma can exacerbate feelings of isolation and prevent individuals from accessing necessary treatment and support.
3. Consequences of Stigma
Barriers to Treatment:

Stigma creates significant barriers to accessing mental health services. Individuals may delay seeking treatment due to fear of judgment or discrimination from healthcare providers or concerns about confidentiality. This delay can worsen symptoms and reduce the effectiveness of interventions.
Social and Economic Impact:

Stigma affects various domains of life, including employment, education, and social relationships. Discrimination in the workplace can lead to job loss, reduced career opportunities, and financial instability. Social stigma may strain family relationships and hinder social integration, contributing to feelings of loneliness and isolation.
4. Addressing Stigma
Education and Awareness:

Increasing public awareness and education about mental health disorders and challenging stereotypes through campaigns, workshops, and media initiatives. Education helps debunk myths, promote understanding, and foster empathy toward individuals living with mental illness.

Policy and Legislation:

Enacting and enforcing anti-discrimination laws and policies that protect the rights of individuals with mental health conditions in employment, housing, healthcare, and public accommodations. Legal protections help ensure equal access to opportunities and promote fair treatment.
Community Support:

Building supportive communities that prioritize mental health awareness and inclusion. Support groups, peer networks, and community organizations play a crucial role in providing emotional support, reducing isolation, and promoting recovery-oriented environments.
Practical Implications
Promoting Resilience: Empowering individuals to challenge stigma, build self-advocacy skills, and seek support from peers and mental health professionals.
Enhancing Treatment Outcomes: Integrating stigma-reduction strategies into mental health interventions to improve treatment adherence, engagement, and overall recovery rates.
Advocacy and Social Change: Collaborating with stakeholders, including policymakers, healthcare providers, educators, and community leaders, to advocate for systemic changes that promote stigma reduction and mental health parity.
Conclusion
Chapter 7 underscores the pervasive impact of stigma on mental health, highlighting its detrimental effects on individuals' well-being, treatment outcomes, and social inclusion. By addressing stigma through education, policy reform, community support, and advocacy efforts, societies can create more inclusive and supportive environments for individuals living with mental illness.

Continue exploring the complexities of stigma and its implications for mental health in "Embracing Social Norms: The Psychology of Human Interaction" by Laurel D. Malvern.

Chapter 8: Foundations of Psychology

Psychology, as a discipline, encompasses the study of human behavior and mental processes. Its foundations lie in understanding how individuals perceive, think, feel, and behave in various contexts. This chapter explores the fundamental principles, theories, and historical developments that have shaped the field of psychology.

1. Introduction to Psychological Theories
Definition and Scope:

Psychology is the scientific study of behavior and mental processes. It seeks to understand the complexities of human cognition, emotions, motivations, and interpersonal interactions through empirical research and theoretical frameworks.
Major Psychological Theories:

Psychoanalytic Theory: Developed by Sigmund Freud, this theory emphasizes unconscious motivations, conflicts, and early childhood experiences in shaping personality and behavior.

Behaviorism: Founded by John B. Watson and later expanded by B.F. Skinner, behaviorism focuses on observable behaviors and the impact of environmental stimuli on learning and behavior.

Cognitive Theory: Introduced by Jean Piaget and others, cognitive theory explores mental processes such as perception, memory, language, and problem-solving, highlighting how these processes influence behavior.

Humanistic Psychology: Advocated by Carl Rogers and Abraham Maslow, humanistic psychology emphasizes personal growth, self-actualization, and the inherent goodness and potential of individuals.

Biological and Evolutionary Psychology: Examines the biological basis of behavior, genetics, brain structure and function, and evolutionary influences on psychological processes and behavior.

2. Historical Context and Evolution

Early Foundations:

Philosophical Roots: Psychology's origins can be traced back to ancient Greek philosophers such as Socrates, Plato, and Aristotle, who pondered the nature of the mind, knowledge, and human behavior.

Structuralism and Functionalism: In the late 19th century, Wilhelm Wundt established the first psychology laboratory, focusing on the study of consciousness and mental structures (structuralism). William James introduced functionalism, emphasizing the adaptive functions of behavior in response to the environment.

Modern Developments:

Growth of Scientific Methods: Psychology evolved into a scientific discipline, embracing rigorous experimental methods, statistical analysis, and empirical research to study human behavior and mental processes.
Diversity of Perspectives: Contemporary psychology encompasses multiple perspectives, including biological, cognitive, behavioral, psychodynamic, humanistic, and socio-cultural approaches, reflecting the complexity of human experience.
3. Key Figures in Psychology and Their Contributions
Founding Figures:

Sigmund Freud: Known for psychoanalytic theory, Freud explored the unconscious mind, defense mechanisms, and the role of early childhood experiences in shaping personality.
B.F. Skinner: A behaviorist, Skinner studied operant conditioning and reinforcement, emphasizing how behavior is shaped by its consequences in the environment.
Jean Piaget: Pioneered cognitive development theory, Piaget explored how children construct knowledge and understand the world through stages of cognitive development.
Carl Rogers: Founder of humanistic psychology, Rogers emphasized self-concept, unconditional positive regard, and the importance of client-centered therapy in facilitating personal growth and self-actualization.
Contemporary Influences:

Neuroscience: Advances in neuroscience have expanded our understanding of brain function, neural pathways, and the biological basis of behavior, contributing to fields such as neuropsychology and cognitive neuroscience.
Cross-Cultural Psychology: Examines cultural influences on psychological processes, values, beliefs, and behaviors, highlighting the diversity of human experience and challenging universal assumptions.
Conclusion

Foundations of psychology provide a comprehensive framework for understanding human behavior, cognition, emotions, and social interactions. By exploring historical developments, major theories, and influential figures in psychology, researchers and practitioners continue to advance our knowledge of the mind and behavior, addressing contemporary challenges and promoting psychological well-being.

This exploration of psychology's foundations sets the stage for deeper insights into human behavior and mental processes in "Embracing Social Norms: The Psychology of Human Interaction" by Laurel D. Malvern.

Chapter 9: Introduction to Psychological Theories

Psychological theories form the foundation of understanding human behavior, cognition, emotions, and interpersonal dynamics. This introduction provides an overview of the major theoretical frameworks that shape the field of psychology, offering insights into how these theories contribute to our understanding of the complexities of the human mind.

Definition and Scope
Psychology: Defined as the scientific study of behavior and mental processes, psychology seeks to explain and predict how individuals perceive, think, feel, and behave in various contexts. It employs empirical research methods, theoretical frameworks, and interdisciplinary approaches to explore the intricacies of human experience.

Major Psychological Theories
Psychoanalytic Theory:

Founder: Sigmund Freud

Key Concepts: Focuses on unconscious motivations, early childhood experiences, and defense mechanisms that shape personality development and behavior. Emphasizes the role of the unconscious mind in influencing thoughts, feelings, and actions.

Behavioral Theory:

Founders: John B. Watson, B.F. Skinner
Key Concepts: Emphasizes observable behaviors and the impact of environmental stimuli on learning, reinforcement, and behavior modification. Behaviorists focus on measurable actions and responses to understand human behavior.

Cognitive Theory:

Founders: Jean Piaget, Albert Bandura
Key Concepts: Examines mental processes such as perception, memory, reasoning, and problem-solving. Cognitive theorists explore how individuals acquire, process, and store information, emphasizing cognition as a key determinant of behavior.

Humanistic Psychology:

Founders: Carl Rogers, Abraham Maslow
Key Concepts: Focuses on human potential, self-actualization, and personal growth. Humanistic psychology emphasizes subjective experiences, free will, and the importance of individual perceptions and choices in shaping behavior.

Biological and Evolutionary Psychology:

Key Concepts: Investigates the biological basis of behavior, genetics, brain structure and function, and evolutionary influences on psychological processes. Explores how physiological factors influence cognition, emotions, and behavior.

Contributions to Understanding Human Behavior

Interdisciplinary Perspectives: Psychological theories draw from diverse disciplines, including neuroscience, sociology, anthropology, and philosophy, to provide comprehensive explanations of human behavior across different levels of analysis.

Practical Applications: Theoretical frameworks inform clinical practice, education, organizational behavior, and public policy, guiding interventions, treatments, and strategies to enhance psychological well-being and promote positive outcomes.

Conclusion
Introduction to psychological theories provides a foundational understanding of the diverse perspectives and methodologies employed in the study of human behavior and mental processes. By examining major theoretical frameworks and their contributions to understanding cognition, emotion, motivation, and social interactions, psychologists continue to advance knowledge and address complex challenges in society.

This introduction sets the stage for deeper exploration into psychological theories in "Embracing Social Norms: The Psychology of Human Interaction" by Laurel D. Malvern, offering insights into the dynamic interplay between theory, research, and application in the field of psychology.

Chapter 10: Historical Context and Evolution of Psychology

Psychology has evolved significantly over centuries, shaped by various philosophical, scientific, and cultural developments. Understanding its historical context provides insights into how the discipline has transformed from philosophical speculation to a scientific field dedicated to studying human behavior, cognition, and mental processes.

Early Foundations
Ancient Philosophical Roots:

Psychology's origins can be traced back to ancient civilizations, where philosophers such as Socrates, Plato, and Aristotle pondered questions about the nature of the mind, consciousness, and human behavior. Their writings laid the groundwork for later psychological inquiries.
Renaissance and Enlightenment Influences:

During the Renaissance and Enlightenment periods (14th to 18th centuries), advances in science, philosophy, and empiricism sparked interest in understanding human nature through empirical observation and reasoning. Thinkers like Descartes, Locke, and Hume explored ideas about the mind, perception, and consciousness.

Emergence of Scientific Psychology
Establishment of the First Psychology Laboratory:

In 1879, Wilhelm Wundt established the first experimental psychology laboratory at the University of Leipzig, Germany. Wundt is often regarded as the father of modern psychology for pioneering experimental methods to study conscious experiences and mental processes.
Structuralism and Functionalism:

Structuralism, advocated by Edward Titchener, focused on analyzing the basic elements of consciousness through introspection. Meanwhile, functionalism, promoted by William James, emphasized the adaptive functions of behavior in response to the environment.
20th Century Developments
Behaviorism:

John B. Watson and B.F. Skinner ushered in the era of behaviorism, which dominated psychology in the early 20th century. Behaviorists focused on observable behaviors and the environmental factors that shape learning, reinforcement, and behavior modification.
Psychoanalysis:

Sigmund Freud introduced psychoanalytic theory, which emphasized unconscious motivations, early childhood experiences, and the dynamic interplay of the id, ego, and superego in shaping personality and behavior. Freud's work had a profound influence on clinical psychology and psychotherapy.
Contemporary Perspectives
Cognitive Revolution:

In the mid-20th century, the cognitive revolution shifted focus to mental processes such as perception, memory, language, and problem-solving. Scholars like Jean Piaget and Albert Bandura contributed to cognitive theories that explored how individuals acquire, process, and store information.
Integration of Biological and Evolutionary Perspectives:

Advances in neuroscience and genetics have expanded understanding of the biological basis of behavior, brain structure and function, and evolutionary influences on psychological processes. Biological and evolutionary psychology examine how physiological factors influence cognition, emotions, and behavior.
Cultural and Global Perspectives
Cross-Cultural Psychology:

Psychology has increasingly embraced cross-cultural perspectives, recognizing the diversity of human experiences, values, and behaviors across different cultures. Cross-cultural psychologists study cultural influences on psychological processes, identity, and social behaviors.
Conclusion
The historical context and evolution of psychology reflect its transformation from philosophical speculation to a rigorous scientific discipline dedicated to understanding human behavior, cognition, and mental health. By examining key milestones, influential figures, and paradigm shifts, psychologists continue to advance knowledge and address complex challenges in society.

Understanding this historical evolution provides a foundational framework for studying psychological theories and practices in contemporary contexts. It underscores the dynamic interplay between historical developments, scientific inquiry, and societal influences in shaping the field of psychology today.

Chapter 11: Key Figures in Psychology and Their Contributions

Psychology, as a discipline, has been shaped by influential figures whose theories and contributions have significantly advanced our understanding of human behavior, cognition, and mental processes. These key figures have introduced groundbreaking ideas, developed influential theories, and pioneered methodologies that continue to shape the field today.

Sigmund Freud (1856-1939)
Contribution: Psychoanalytic Theory

Theory: Freud developed psychoanalytic theory, which posits that unconscious drives and early childhood experiences influence personality development and behavior. He introduced concepts such as the id, ego, superego, defense mechanisms, and psychosexual stages of development.

Impact: Freud's work laid the foundation for psychoanalysis, a therapeutic approach that explores unconscious conflicts and aims to bring repressed emotions and memories into conscious awareness. His theories influenced clinical psychology, personality theory, and cultural studies.
Wilhelm Wundt (1832-1920)
Contribution: Establishing Psychology as a Science

Achievement: Wundt is often regarded as the father of experimental psychology for establishing the first psychology laboratory at the University of Leipzig in 1879.
Methodology: He pioneered introspection as a method to study conscious experiences, aiming to break down mental processes into basic components. Wundt's work laid the groundwork for structuralism and contributed to the emergence of psychology as a scientific discipline.
John B. Watson (1878-1958) and B.F. Skinner (1904-1990)
Contribution: Behaviorism

Theory: Watson and Skinner were pivotal figures in behaviorism, which emphasizes observable behaviors and the influence of environmental stimuli on learning and behavior.
Behaviorism's Impact: Watson's famous "Little Albert" experiment demonstrated classical conditioning, while Skinner's work on operant conditioning and reinforcement principles shaped behaviorist principles in education, therapy, and behavioral modification.
Jean Piaget (1896-1980)
Contribution: Cognitive Development Theory

Theory: Piaget proposed a stage theory of cognitive development, outlining how children's thinking evolves through stages from infancy to adolescence. His work emphasized the role of schemas, assimilation, accommodation, and the importance of active exploration in learning.

Legacy: Piaget's theories have influenced educational practices, child development research, and our understanding of cognitive processes in both children and adults.
Carl Rogers (1902-1987)
Contribution: Humanistic Psychology

Theory: Rogers pioneered humanistic psychology, emphasizing personal growth, self-actualization, and the innate drive towards fulfillment and authenticity.
Client-Centered Therapy: He introduced client-centered therapy, which focuses on creating a supportive therapeutic environment where clients can explore their feelings, thoughts, and experiences without judgment. Rogers emphasized empathy, unconditional positive regard, and authenticity in therapeutic relationships.
Albert Bandura (1925-present)
Contribution: Social Learning Theory

Theory: Bandura's social learning theory integrates cognitive and behavioral approaches, emphasizing the role of observation, imitation, and modeling in learning and behavior.
Bobo Doll Experiment: His research, including the Bobo doll experiment, demonstrated how children learn aggressive behaviors through observational learning and modeling.
Impact: Bandura's work has influenced social psychology, education, and theories of behavior change, highlighting the importance of cognitive factors and social influences in shaping behavior.
Conclusion

These key figures in psychology have made profound contributions to the field, shaping theoretical frameworks, research methodologies, and therapeutic approaches that continue to inform psychological practice and research today. Their work has not only expanded our understanding of human behavior and mental processes but also paved the way for diverse perspectives and interdisciplinary collaborations within psychology.

Chapter 12: The Nature of Relationships

Relationships are fundamental to human existence, encompassing various types of connections that individuals form with others. Understanding the nature of relationships involves exploring their dynamics, functions, and psychological underpinnings across different contexts.

Types of Relationships: Familial, Romantic, Platonic
Familial Relationships:

Definition: These relationships include those with parents, siblings, extended family members, and caregivers. They are typically characterized by blood ties, shared history, and a sense of kinship.

Functions: Familial relationships provide emotional support, socialization, and identity formation. They often play a crucial role in shaping an individual's values, beliefs, and cultural practices.
Romantic Relationships:

Definition: Romantic relationships involve emotional and physical intimacy between partners who share romantic feelings and commitment. They can range from dating relationships to long-term partnerships and marriages.
Functions: Romantic relationships fulfill emotional needs for intimacy, companionship, love, and sexual expression. They contribute to personal growth, mutual support, and the formation of shared goals and aspirations.
Platonic Relationships:

Definition: These relationships involve deep emotional bonds, trust, and camaraderie between friends and acquaintances. They do not typically involve romantic or sexual attraction.
Functions: Platonic relationships provide social support, companionship, and opportunities for shared interests and activities. They contribute to emotional well-being, personal development, and a sense of belonging.
The Psychology of Attachment
Attachment Theory:

Concept: Developed by John Bowlby and Mary Ainsworth, attachment theory explores how early interactions with caregivers shape patterns of attachment and influence relationships throughout life.
Attachment Styles: Secure, anxious-preoccupied, dismissive-avoidant, and fearful-avoidant attachment styles reflect individuals' beliefs about themselves and others in relationships.

Impact: Attachment styles influence how individuals perceive intimacy, manage emotions in relationships, and seek support during times of stress.

Dynamics and Maintenance of Healthy Relationships
Communication: Effective communication is essential for maintaining healthy relationships. It involves expressing thoughts, feelings, and needs clearly, actively listening to others, and resolving conflicts constructively.

Trust and Commitment: Trust is the foundation of healthy relationships, built through honesty, reliability, and mutual respect. Commitment involves dedication to the relationship's growth and well-being over time.

Conflict Resolution: Addressing conflicts respectfully and collaboratively is crucial for relationship maintenance. Techniques such as active listening, compromise, and problem-solving help partners navigate disagreements and strengthen their bond.

Conclusion
The nature of relationships encompasses a complex interplay of emotional, social, and cognitive factors that shape human interactions and connections. By exploring the dynamics, functions, and psychological processes underlying familial, romantic, and platonic relationships, psychologists deepen our understanding of interpersonal dynamics and the ways individuals form, maintain, and nurture meaningful connections throughout their lives. Understanding these aspects enhances our ability to cultivate and sustain healthy, fulfilling relationships in various social contexts.

Chapter 13: Types of Relationships: Familial, Romantic, Platonic

Relationships are fundamental to human experience, providing individuals with social connections, emotional support, and a sense of belonging. Understanding the different types of relationships sheds light on the diverse ways humans interact and form bonds with others.

Familial Relationships
Definition: Familial relationships are based on blood ties, legal bonds (such as adoption), or cultural and communal connections. They typically involve close and enduring relationships with relatives.

Characteristics:

Blood Ties: Familial relationships are often characterized by biological connections, such as parent-child, sibling-sibling, and extended family relationships.
Shared History: These relationships are rooted in shared experiences, traditions, and cultural practices that contribute to a sense of identity and belonging within the family unit.
Supportive Networks: Familial relationships provide emotional support, practical assistance, and socialization opportunities that contribute to individual development and well-being.
Functions:

Emotional Support: Family members offer comfort, empathy, and encouragement during challenging times, fostering emotional resilience and security.
Socialization: Families play a crucial role in transmitting values, norms, and traditions across generations, shaping individuals' beliefs, behaviors, and identities.
Identity Formation: Family relationships contribute to the development of self-concept and personal identity through interactions and roles within the family structure.
Romantic Relationships
Definition: Romantic relationships involve emotional and physical intimacy between partners who share romantic attraction, affection, and commitment.

Characteristics:

Intimacy: Romantic relationships prioritize emotional closeness, shared experiences, and physical affection between partners.
Commitment: Partners in romantic relationships often express mutual dedication, exclusivity, and long-term goals for the relationship's growth and stability.

Sexual Expression: Romantic relationships include sexual intimacy as a component of bonding and connection between partners.
Functions:

Companionship and Emotional Fulfillment: Romantic relationships fulfill individuals' needs for companionship, emotional support, and validation of self-worth.
Personal Growth: Partners support each other's personal development, goals, and aspirations, fostering mutual growth and self-discovery.
Family Building: Romantic relationships may lead to marriage or cohabitation, with the potential for starting a family and parenting together.
Platonic Relationships
Definition: Platonic relationships are non-romantic and non-sexual friendships characterized by emotional closeness, mutual respect, and shared interests.

Characteristics:

Friendship: Platonic relationships are built on friendship bonds that prioritize companionship, trust, and loyalty without romantic or sexual attraction.
Emotional Support: Friends in platonic relationships provide emotional encouragement, understanding, and empathy during both joyful and challenging life events.
Shared Activities: Platonic relationships involve shared interests, hobbies, and experiences that strengthen the bond between friends.
Functions:

Social Support: Platonic relationships offer social companionship, camaraderie, and a sense of belonging within peer groups and social circles.

Conflict Resolution: Friends in platonic relationships navigate conflicts, disagreements, and misunderstandings through open communication and mutual respect.

Personal Enrichment: Platonic relationships contribute to personal happiness, well-being, and a sense of community through meaningful connections and shared experiences.

Conclusion

Understanding the diverse types of relationships—familial, romantic, and platonic—provides insights into the multifaceted ways humans connect, interact, and support one another across various social contexts. Each type of relationship offers unique opportunities for emotional fulfillment, personal growth, and social connectedness, enriching individuals' lives and contributing to their overall well-being and happiness. Recognizing and nurturing these relationships enhances interpersonal skills, strengthens social bonds, and fosters a sense of community and belonging in diverse communities and cultures worldwide.

Chapter 14: The Psychology of Attachment

Attachment theory, developed by John Bowlby and expanded upon by Mary Ainsworth and others, provides a framework for understanding how early experiences with caregivers shape human development and influence relationships throughout life. Attachment theory emphasizes the importance of close emotional bonds, or attachments, between infants and caregivers as foundational to psychological development.

Key Concepts in Attachment Theory
1. Attachment Styles:

Attachment styles are patterns of relational behavior that develop in response to early caregiving experiences. The main attachment styles identified by researchers are:
Secure Attachment: Children with secure attachment styles feel safe and confident in their caregivers' availability and responsiveness. They explore their environment freely and seek comfort from caregivers when needed.
Anxious-Preoccupied Attachment: Individuals with this style may feel insecure about their worthiness of love and attention, often seeking reassurance and approval from others.

Dismissive-Avoidant Attachment: Individuals with this style may avoid intimacy and emotional closeness, preferring independence and self-reliance.

Fearful-Avoidant Attachment: This style combines elements of both anxious and dismissive attachment, where individuals desire closeness but fear rejection or abandonment.

2. Internal Working Models:

Internal working models are mental representations or schemas formed based on early attachment experiences. These models influence how individuals perceive themselves, others, and relationships, guiding expectations and behaviors in future relationships.

Positive early experiences with caregivers tend to foster secure attachment and positive internal working models, while inconsistent or negative experiences can lead to insecure attachment styles and negative internal working models.

3. Impact on Development and Relationships:

Attachment theory suggests that early attachment experiences lay the foundation for emotional regulation, social competence, and relationship satisfaction throughout life. Securely attached individuals often exhibit greater resilience, empathy, and emotional intelligence, whereas insecurely attached individuals may struggle with trust, intimacy, and self-esteem in relationships.

Applications of Attachment Theory

1. Parenting and Caregiving:

Attachment theory informs parenting practices by highlighting the importance of responsive and nurturing caregiving to promote secure attachment bonds with children. Parents can foster secure attachment by being emotionally available, responsive to their child's needs, and providing a safe and supportive environment.

2. Therapy and Counseling:

Attachment-based therapies help individuals understand and modify their attachment patterns to develop more secure and satisfying relationships.

Therapists may use techniques such as reflective listening, exploring early attachment experiences, and promoting emotional attunement to support clients in forming healthier relationship dynamics.

3. Romantic Relationships:

Attachment theory offers insights into adult romantic relationships by examining how attachment styles influence partner selection, communication patterns, and relationship satisfaction.

Couples therapy may focus on enhancing emotional attunement, addressing attachment-related insecurities, and promoting secure base behaviors in intimate relationships.

Conclusion

The psychology of attachment underscores the significance of early caregiving experiences in shaping emotional development, interpersonal relationships, and psychological well-being across the lifespan. By understanding attachment styles, internal working models, and their implications for personal growth and relationship dynamics, psychologists and individuals can cultivate secure attachments, promote resilience, and foster healthier relationships in diverse social contexts. Attachment theory continues to inform research, clinical practice, and interventions aimed at supporting individuals in developing meaningful connections and achieving emotional fulfillment throughout their lives.

Chapter 15: Dynamics and Maintenance of Healthy Relationships

Healthy relationships are characterized by mutual respect, trust, effective communication, and emotional support. Understanding the dynamics and principles that contribute to maintaining these relationships is crucial for fostering intimacy, resolving conflicts, and sustaining long-term connections.

Dynamics of Healthy Relationships
1. Communication:

Effective Communication: Healthy relationships thrive on open, honest, and respectful communication. Partners listen actively, express their thoughts and feelings clearly, and validate each other's perspectives.
Nonverbal Communication: Nonverbal cues such as eye contact, body language, and facial expressions also play a significant role in conveying emotions and understanding in relationships.
2. Trust and Respect:

Trust: Trust is the foundation of healthy relationships, built over time through consistent actions, reliability, and honesty. Partners trust each other's intentions, decisions, and commitments.

Respect: Mutual respect involves valuing each other's opinions, boundaries, and autonomy. Partners show respect by honoring differences, seeking consent, and avoiding demeaning or dismissive behavior.

3. Emotional Support:

Empathy and Understanding: Partners in healthy relationships demonstrate empathy by understanding each other's emotions, perspectives, and experiences. They offer emotional support during both joyful and challenging times.

Validation and Affirmation: Validating each other's feelings and affirming their strengths and efforts fosters a sense of security and emotional closeness in relationships.

Maintenance of Healthy Relationships

1. Conflict Resolution:

Constructive Conflict: Conflicts are inevitable in relationships, but healthy couples resolve them through constructive communication, compromise, and problem-solving.

Active Listening: Partners practice active listening by focusing on understanding rather than reacting defensively. They seek clarification, express empathy, and avoid blame or criticism.

2. Quality Time and Shared Activities:

Quality Time: Spending meaningful time together strengthens emotional bonds and connection. Partners engage in activities they both enjoy, fostering positive experiences and shared memories.

Shared Goals and Interests: Aligning goals and interests encourages collaboration, mutual support, and a sense of partnership in achieving common objectives.

3. Continued Growth and Adaptation:

Individual Growth: Healthy relationships support individual growth and personal development. Partners encourage each other's aspirations, hobbies, and self-improvement efforts.
Adaptability: Relationships evolve over time, requiring flexibility and adaptability to navigate life changes, transitions, and challenges together.
Strategies for Maintenance
1. Regular Check-Ins: Partners engage in regular conversations to assess relationship satisfaction, discuss concerns, and identify areas for improvement.
2. Relationship Rituals: Establishing rituals such as date nights, shared hobbies, or daily affirmations reinforces connection and commitment.
3. Seeking Support: Seeking guidance from couples therapy or relationship counseling can provide tools, insights, and strategies for enhancing relationship dynamics and resolving conflicts effectively.

Conclusion
Understanding the dynamics and maintenance of healthy relationships involves cultivating effective communication, building trust and respect, providing emotional support, and navigating conflicts constructively. By prioritizing these principles and practices, individuals can nurture fulfilling, resilient, and mutually satisfying relationships that contribute to their emotional well-being and overall quality of life. Continuous effort, mutual understanding, and commitment to growth are essential for sustaining healthy relationships over time.

Chapter 16: Behavior – Understanding Actions

Behavior is a fundamental aspect of human interaction and communication, encompassing a wide range of actions, responses, and expressions that individuals exhibit in various contexts. Understanding the factors that influence behavior provides insights into human cognition, emotions, social interactions, and decision-making processes.

Factors Influencing Behavior
1. Psychological Factors:

Cognition and Perception: How individuals perceive and interpret situations, events, and stimuli influences their behavioral responses. Cognitive processes such as attention, memory, and decision-making shape behavioral choices.
Emotions: Emotional experiences and states affect behavior by influencing motivations, responses to stressors, and social interactions. Emotion regulation strategies impact how individuals express and manage their feelings in different contexts.
2. Social and Cultural Factors:

Social Norms and Expectations: Social norms prescribe appropriate behaviors within a specific cultural or societal context. Conforming to social norms reinforces group cohesion, acceptance, and conformity to established behavioral standards.

Social Influence: Peer pressure, social roles, and group dynamics influence behavior by shaping attitudes, beliefs, and behaviors through social interaction and conformity.

3. Environmental and Situational Factors:

Physical Environment: Environmental cues, settings, and conditions impact behavior by providing opportunities, constraints, and stimuli that guide actions and decisions.

Situational Context: Immediate circumstances, events, and interpersonal dynamics influence behavioral responses, adaptive strategies, and problem-solving approaches.

Behavioral Theories and Applications

1. Learning Theories:

Behaviorism: Behaviorist theories emphasize observable behaviors, reinforcement, and conditioning processes that shape behavior through rewards, punishments, and environmental stimuli.

Social Learning Theory: Social learning theory posits that behavior is acquired and modified through observational learning, modeling, and reinforcement of behaviors observed in others.

2. Motivational Theories:

Hierarchy of Needs (Maslow): Maslow's hierarchy of needs suggests that human behavior is driven by innate needs for physiological survival, safety, belongingness, esteem, and self-actualization.

Expectancy Theory: Expectancy theory examines how individual expectations of outcomes, effort-performance relationships, and valence influence motivational behaviors and goal-directed actions.

3. Cognitive Theories:

Cognitive-Behavioral Theory: Cognitive-behavioral theory integrates cognitive processes (thoughts, beliefs, perceptions) and behavioral responses, emphasizing the role of cognitive restructuring in modifying behaviors and emotional responses.

Attribution Theory: Attribution theory explores how individuals interpret and attribute causes to their own and others' behaviors, influencing self-perception, social interactions, and emotional responses.

Behavior Modification Techniques

1. Reinforcement: Positive reinforcement involves rewarding desired behaviors to increase their occurrence, while negative reinforcement removes aversive stimuli to reinforce adaptive behaviors.

2. Punishment: Punishment discourages undesirable behaviors through the application of aversive consequences, reducing the likelihood of their repetition.

3. Extinction: Extinction reduces the frequency of undesirable behaviors by removing reinforcement or consequences previously reinforcing the behavior.

Conclusion

Understanding behavior involves exploring the complex interplay of psychological, social, cultural, and environmental factors that shape human actions, decisions, and interactions. Behavioral theories and applications provide frameworks for analyzing behavior, predicting outcomes, and implementing interventions to promote adaptive behaviors, personal growth, and social well-being. By enhancing understanding of behavior, individuals and practitioners can cultivate self-awareness, improve interpersonal relationships, and facilitate positive changes in behavior across diverse contexts and settings.

Chaoter 17: Behavioral Theories

1. Behaviorism:

Key Concepts: Behaviorism, pioneered by psychologists such as B.F. Skinner and John B. Watson, focuses on observable behaviors rather than internal mental processes. It suggests that behaviors are shaped by environmental factors through processes of reinforcement and conditioning.

Applications: Behaviorism is applied in various fields, including education, therapy, and organizational behavior. In education, teachers use principles of behaviorism to reinforce desired behaviors through rewards and consequences. In therapy, behavioral techniques like systematic desensitization and token economies are used to treat phobias and modify maladaptive behaviors. In organizational settings, behaviorism informs management practices by emphasizing incentives and consequences to motivate employees.
2. Social Learning Theory:

Key Concepts: Social learning theory, developed by Albert Bandura, posits that individuals learn behaviors through observation, imitation, and modeling of others. It emphasizes the role of cognitive processes in learning and behavior change, including attention, retention, reproduction, and motivation.
Applications: Social learning theory is applied in education and therapy to teach new skills and behaviors. In education, modeling behaviors and providing opportunities for observational learning can enhance learning outcomes. In therapy, modeling positive behaviors and providing social support can facilitate behavior change and skill acquisition.
3. Cognitive-Behavioral Theory:

Key Concepts: Cognitive-behavioral theory integrates cognitive processes (thoughts, beliefs, attitudes) with behavioral principles. It suggests that cognitive interpretations of events influence emotions and behaviors. Behavioral change occurs through cognitive restructuring, which involves identifying and modifying negative or irrational thoughts.

Applications: Cognitive-behavioral therapy (CBT) is widely used to treat various mental health conditions, including anxiety disorders, depression, and substance abuse. CBT techniques such as cognitive restructuring, behavioral activation, and exposure therapy help individuals change maladaptive behaviors and improve coping skills.
Applications of Behavioral Theories
1. Education:

Classroom Management: Teachers use behaviorist principles to establish classroom rules, reinforce positive behaviors, and manage student behavior effectively.
Learning Strategies: Social learning theory informs instructional practices by incorporating modeling and observational learning to teach complex skills and behaviors.
2. Clinical Psychology:

Behavioral Interventions: Behaviorism and CBT are applied in clinical settings to address behavioral problems, improve coping skills, and treat mental health disorders through structured interventions.
Behavior Modification: Techniques like reinforcement, punishment, and extinction are used to modify behaviors and promote adaptive responses in therapeutic contexts.
3. Organizational Behavior:

Performance Management: Managers apply behaviorist principles to motivate employees, shape organizational culture, and enhance performance through rewards, recognition, and feedback.
Training and Development: Social learning theory informs training programs by emphasizing role modeling, peer learning, and experiential learning to develop skills and competencies.
Conclusion

Behavioral theories provide valuable frameworks for understanding human behavior, learning processes, and behavior change mechanisms across diverse contexts. By applying these theories, practitioners in psychology, education, and organizational behavior can design effective interventions, promote positive behaviors, and facilitate personal and professional growth. Understanding behavioral theories enhances our ability to predict and influence behaviors, ultimately contributing to individual well-being and societal development.

Chapter 18: Factors Influencing Behavior

1. Psychological Factors:

Cognition and Perception: How individuals perceive and interpret their environment influences their behavioral responses. Cognitive processes such as attention, memory, decision-making, and problem-solving play a significant role in shaping behavior.
Emotions: Emotional experiences and states affect behavior by influencing motivations, responses to stressors, and interpersonal interactions. Emotional regulation strategies impact how individuals express and manage their feelings in various contexts.
2. Social Factors:

Social Norms: Social norms dictate acceptable behaviors within a specific cultural or societal context. Conforming to social norms reinforces group cohesion, acceptance, and adherence to established behavioral standards.
Social Influence: Peer pressure, social roles, group dynamics, and interpersonal relationships influence behavior by shaping attitudes, beliefs, and actions through social interaction and conformity.
3. Cultural Factors:

Cultural Values: Cultural beliefs, values, traditions, and norms shape behavioral expectations and practices within different cultural contexts. Cultural diversity influences behaviors related to communication styles, social interactions, and decision-making processes.

Acculturation: Individuals navigate between their cultural heritage and the dominant culture, impacting their behaviors, identities, and adaptation strategies within multicultural societies.

4. Environmental and Situational Factors:

Physical Environment: Environmental factors such as geography, climate, architecture, and urban design influence behavior by providing opportunities, constraints, and stimuli that guide actions and decisions.

Situational Context: Immediate circumstances, events, and interpersonal dynamics influence behavioral responses, adaptive strategies, and problem-solving approaches in specific situations.

Applications in Understanding Behavior

1. Psychology:

Behavioral Assessment: Psychologists assess the influence of psychological factors on behavior through cognitive assessments, personality tests, and behavioral observations to understand motivations and decision-making processes.

Therapeutic Interventions: Behavioral therapies, such as cognitive-behavioral therapy (CBT), address maladaptive behaviors by modifying cognitive distortions, teaching coping skills, and promoting behavioral change.

2. Sociology and Anthropology:

Social Structures: Sociologists study how social structures, institutions, and group dynamics influence collective behaviors, social movements, and societal norms within communities.

Cultural Anthropology: Anthropologists examine how cultural beliefs, rituals, and practices shape individual and collective behaviors across diverse cultural contexts.

3. Public Policy and Education:

Behavioral Economics: Economists apply behavioral insights to design policies that promote desired behaviors, such as saving money, environmental conservation, and healthy lifestyle choices.

Educational Strategies: Educators use behavioral theories to develop effective teaching strategies, classroom management techniques, and learning interventions that accommodate diverse learning styles and behavioral needs.

Conclusion

Behavior is influenced by a multifaceted interplay of psychological, social, cultural, and environmental factors. By understanding these influences, psychologists, sociologists, educators, policymakers, and other professionals can better predict, explain, and intervene in behaviors to promote positive outcomes and enhance individual and societal well-being. Continued research and application of behavioral theories contribute to advancing knowledge, improving interventions, and fostering adaptive behaviors across diverse contexts and populations.

Chapter 19: Behavior Modification Techniques

1. Reinforcement:

Positive Reinforcement: Involves presenting a positive stimulus (reward) immediately following a desired behavior to increase the likelihood of that behavior recurring in the future. For example, praising a student for completing homework on time to encourage consistent study habits. Negative Reinforcement: Removes or avoids an aversive stimulus upon the occurrence of a desired behavior, which strengthens the likelihood of the behavior being repeated. An example is allowing a child to skip chores after completing homework, reinforcing compliance with academic responsibilities.
2. Punishment:

Positive Punishment: Introduces an aversive stimulus (punishment) following an undesired behavior to decrease the likelihood of that behavior occurring again. This can include reprimanding a child for disruptive behavior in class. Negative Punishment: Involves removing a positive stimulus (taking away privileges) following an undesired behavior to decrease the likelihood of that behavior in the future. For instance, taking away a teenager's driving privileges for breaking curfew.
3. Extinction:

Extinction: Involves withholding reinforcement or consequences that previously reinforced a behavior, thereby reducing the occurrence of that behavior over time. For example, ignoring attention-seeking behavior in a child may eventually lead to the extinction of that behavior if it no longer results in attention.
4. Token Economy:

Token Economy: Utilizes tokens or points as secondary reinforcers that can be exchanged for desired rewards or privileges. This technique is often used in educational settings and institutional environments to encourage positive behaviors consistently over time. For instance, students earn tokens for completing assignments or exhibiting good behavior, which can be exchanged for extra recess time or other rewards.
5. Shaping:

Shaping: Involves reinforcing successive approximations of a target behavior until the desired behavior is achieved. This technique breaks down complex behaviors into smaller, manageable steps, reinforcing each step toward the ultimate goal. For example, teaching a child to tie shoes by initially reinforcing any attempt to touch or hold the shoelaces, gradually shaping toward tying a complete knot.
Applications of Behavior Modification
1. Clinical Psychology:

Behavioral Therapy: Therapists use behavior modification techniques, such as reinforcement and extinction, to treat behavioral disorders (e.g., phobias, obsessive-compulsive disorder) and promote adaptive behaviors and coping strategies.
2. Education:

Classroom Management: Teachers employ behavior modification techniques to establish rules, reinforce positive behaviors, and manage student conduct effectively in educational settings.

Special Education: Behavior modification techniques are used to support students with behavioral challenges or learning disabilities by teaching adaptive behaviors and reducing disruptive behaviors.

3. Organizational Behavior Management:

Performance Management: Managers use behavior modification techniques to motivate employees, enhance productivity, and promote desirable workplace behaviors through rewards, recognition, and feedback.

4. Parenting and Child Development:

Parenting Strategies: Parents apply behavior modification techniques to encourage desired behaviors (e.g., chores, study habits) and discourage undesirable behaviors (e.g., tantrums, aggression) through consistent reinforcement and consequences.

Conclusion

Behavior modification techniques are effective tools for promoting positive behaviors, reducing maladaptive behaviors, and facilitating behavior change across diverse populations and settings. By understanding the principles of reinforcement, punishment, extinction, token economies, and shaping, practitioners can design tailored interventions that enhance learning, improve mental health outcomes, optimize organizational performance, and support personal development. Continued research and application of behavior modification contribute to advancing behavioral sciences and improving outcomes in behavioral interventions and therapies.

Chapter 20: Emotions: The Heart of Human Experience

1. Theories of Emotion:

James-Lange Theory: Proposed by William James and Carl Lange, this theory suggests that emotions arise from physiological responses to stimuli. For example, feeling fear after experiencing a racing heart and sweaty palms in a threatening situation.

Cannon-Bard Theory: Walter Cannon and Philip Bard proposed that emotions and physiological responses occur simultaneously yet independently in response to stimuli. For instance, feeling fear and experiencing physiological arousal concurrently upon encountering a threat.

Schachter-Singer Two-Factor Theory: Stanley Schachter and Jerome Singer's theory posits that emotions result from a combination of physiological arousal and cognitive appraisal of situational cues. This theory emphasizes the role of cognitive interpretations in emotional experiences.

2. Emotional Regulation:

Definition: Emotional regulation refers to the ability to manage and modify emotional experiences, expressions, and responses effectively. It involves strategies to enhance positive emotions, reduce negative emotions, and maintain emotional stability across different situations.

Strategies: Techniques such as cognitive reappraisal (reinterpreting situations to alter emotional responses), expressive suppression (inhibiting emotional expressions), and mindfulness (non-judgmental awareness of present emotions) are used to regulate emotions adaptively.
3. The Interplay Between Emotion and Cognition:

Emotion-Cognition Interaction: Emotions influence cognitive processes, such as attention, memory, decision-making, and problem-solving. For instance, positive emotions can enhance creativity and broaden cognitive perspectives, while negative emotions may narrow focus and lead to risk aversion.
Cognitive Appraisal: Individuals' subjective evaluations (appraisals) of events or situations shape emotional responses. Primary appraisals assess relevance to goals or well-being, while secondary appraisals evaluate coping resources and potential strategies.
4. Importance in Human Behavior:

Motivation: Emotions motivate adaptive behaviors by directing attention towards significant stimuli, guiding decision-making, and promoting goal pursuit. For example, feeling joy may encourage social engagement and exploration, while fear motivates defensive or avoidant responses.
Social Functioning: Emotions facilitate social interactions by conveying information about individuals' states, intentions, and relational dynamics. Empathy, compassion, and emotional contagion enhance interpersonal connections and cooperation within social groups.
Applications in Psychology and Everyday Life
1. Clinical Psychology:

Emotion-Focused Therapy: Therapeutic approaches focus on identifying and processing emotions to promote emotional awareness, regulation, and resilience in individuals experiencing mood disorders or trauma.

2. Education:

Social-Emotional Learning (SEL): Educational programs integrate emotional awareness, empathy, and interpersonal skills to support students' emotional development, academic achievement, and positive behavior.
3. Workplace Dynamics:

Emotional Intelligence: Organizational practices emphasize emotional intelligence (EQ) competencies, such as self-awareness, social awareness, self-management, and relationship management, to enhance leadership, teamwork, and employee well-being.
4. Personal Growth and Well-being:

Mindfulness Practices: Techniques like meditation and deep breathing promote emotional regulation, stress reduction, and overall mental well-being by cultivating present-moment awareness and acceptance of emotional experiences.
Conclusion
Emotions serve as integral components of human experience, influencing cognitive processes, social interactions, and adaptive behaviors across diverse contexts. Understanding theories of emotion, strategies for emotional regulation, and the interplay between emotion and cognition enhances personal growth, interpersonal relationships, and psychological well-being. Continued research in emotional psychology contributes to advancing therapeutic interventions, educational practices, and organizational strategies that promote emotional awareness, resilience, and effective emotional expression in individuals and communities.

Chapter 21: Theories of Emotion

1. James-Lange Theory:

Overview: Proposed independently by psychologist William James and physiologist Carl Lange in the late 19th century. This theory suggests that emotions are the result of physiological reactions to stimuli in the environment. Mechanism: According to the James-Lange theory, specific physiological changes (such as increased heart rate, sweaty palms) precede and cause emotional experiences. For example, encountering a bear in the woods triggers physiological arousal (racing heart, trembling), leading to the emotion of fear.
2. Cannon-Bard Theory:

Overview: Developed by Walter Cannon and Philip Bard in the early 20th century as a critique of the James-Lange theory. It posits that emotional experiences and physiological responses occur simultaneously but independently in response to stimuli.
Mechanism: According to this theory, encountering a threatening stimulus simultaneously triggers both physiological responses (such as increased heart rate) and emotional experiences (such as fear). These responses are independent but occur simultaneously, suggesting a more integrated response compared to the James-Lange model.
3. Schachter-Singer Two-Factor Theory:

Overview: Proposed by Stanley Schachter and Jerome Singer in 1962, this theory integrates physiological arousal and cognitive appraisal to explain emotional experiences.
Mechanism: According to the two-factor theory, emotions are the result of physiological arousal and a cognitive interpretation (appraisal) of the situation. Physiological arousal is seen as a nonspecific state that can be interpreted in different ways depending on the context and cognitive appraisal. For instance, encountering a potential threat (physiological arousal) may lead to fear if the situation is appraised as dangerous or excitement if perceived as thrilling.
4. Lazarus' Cognitive Mediational Theory:

Overview: Developed by Richard Lazarus in the 1960s, this theory emphasizes the role of cognitive appraisal in the experience and regulation of emotions.
Mechanism: Lazarus proposed that emotions arise from the cognitive appraisal of an event or situation, focusing on whether the event is perceived as beneficial or harmful to one's well-being. Primary appraisal involves evaluating the significance of an event to one's goals or well-being, while secondary appraisal assesses one's ability to cope with the event. Emotions are thus viewed as the result of these appraisals, influencing subsequent emotional responses and behaviors.
5. Facial Feedback Hypothesis:

Overview: This hypothesis suggests that facial expressions not only reflect emotional experiences but also contribute to the experience and intensity of emotions.

Mechanism: According to the facial feedback hypothesis, facial muscles and expressions send signals to the brain that influence emotional experiences. For example, smiling can enhance feelings of happiness, while frowning can intensify feelings of sadness or anger. This feedback loop between facial expressions and emotional experiences underscores the bidirectional relationship between emotional expression and experience.

Practical Implications and Applications

Clinical Psychology: Understanding theories of emotion informs therapeutic interventions, such as emotion-focused therapy, which helps individuals identify and regulate emotions effectively.

Education: Educational strategies, including social-emotional learning programs, incorporate theories of emotion to promote emotional intelligence, empathy, and interpersonal skills among students.

Workplace Dynamics: Organizational practices utilize theories of emotion to foster emotional intelligence and effective leadership, enhancing team collaboration and employee well-being.

Personal Development: Applying theories of emotion helps individuals cultivate self-awareness, manage stress, and enhance emotional resilience in various life situations.

Conclusion

Theories of emotion provide diverse perspectives on the complex mechanisms underlying emotional experiences, offering insights into the interplay between physiological processes, cognitive appraisal, and behavioral responses. By understanding these theories, psychologists, educators, and individuals can better comprehend and navigate the intricate landscape of human emotions, fostering emotional well-being, interpersonal relationships, and overall psychological health.

Chapter 22: Emotional Regulation: Definition and Components

1. Definition: Emotional regulation encompasses various processes and strategies individuals use to monitor, evaluate, and modify their emotional reactions. It involves both conscious and unconscious efforts to manage emotional intensity, duration, and expression in response to internal and external stimuli.

2. Components of Emotional Regulation:

Awareness and Identification: The first step in emotional regulation involves recognizing and labeling one's emotional experiences accurately. This awareness helps individuals understand the triggers and context influencing their emotions.

Appraisal and Interpretation: Cognitive appraisal involves evaluating the significance of emotional stimuli and their implications for personal goals, values, and well-being. Positive appraisals can enhance positive emotions, while negative interpretations may exacerbate negative emotional responses.

Response Modulation: Once emotions are identified and appraised, individuals can employ strategies to modulate emotional responses effectively. This may include altering thoughts (cognitive reappraisal), behaviors (emotion-focused coping), or physiological arousal (deep breathing, relaxation techniques).

Importance of Emotional Regulation
1. Psychological Well-being:

Stress Management: Effective emotional regulation helps individuals cope with stressors and challenges, reducing the impact of negative emotions on mental health. It promotes resilience in navigating adversity and maintaining psychological equilibrium.

Mood Regulation: Regulating emotions allows individuals to modulate mood states, promoting positive emotional experiences and reducing prolonged negative affectivity. This contributes to greater emotional stability and overall subjective well-being.

2. Interpersonal Relationships:

Enhanced Communication: Emotionally regulated individuals are better equipped to express emotions constructively and respond empathetically to others' emotional cues. This fosters supportive relationships, empathy, and effective communication.

Conflict Resolution: Effective emotional regulation mitigates interpersonal conflicts by promoting calm, rational responses and reducing emotional reactivity. It facilitates conflict resolution through empathetic understanding and collaborative problem-solving.

3. Cognitive Functioning:

Decision-Making: Emotional regulation facilitates sound decision-making by minimizing the influence of transient emotional states on judgment and reasoning processes. It allows for more thoughtful, goal-oriented choices aligned with long-term objectives.

Attention and Concentration: Regulating emotions prevents emotional distractions and enhances focus on tasks, improving cognitive performance and productivity in academic, professional, and personal domains.

Applications in Different Contexts
1. Clinical Settings:

Therapeutic Interventions: Techniques such as cognitive-behavioral therapy (CBT) integrate emotional regulation strategies to treat mood disorders, anxiety, trauma-related symptoms, and personality disorders.
2. Educational Environments:

Social-Emotional Learning (SEL): Schools incorporate emotional regulation skills into curricula to promote emotional intelligence, self-management, and positive social behaviors among students.
3. Workplace Strategies:

Leadership and Team Dynamics: Organizational training programs emphasize emotional intelligence competencies to enhance leadership effectiveness, team cohesion, and employee resilience in high-stress environments.
Conclusion
Emotional regulation is a foundational skill that underpins adaptive functioning, psychological resilience, and interpersonal relationships across various life domains. By cultivating awareness, employing effective strategies, and integrating emotional regulation into daily practices, individuals enhance their emotional well-being, interpersonal effectiveness, and overall quality of life. Continued research and application of emotional regulation principles contribute to promoting mental health, fostering positive social interactions, and optimizing personal and professional success.

Chapter 23: Understanding Emotion and Cognition

1. Definition and Components:

Emotion: Emotion refers to subjective feelings that are typically accompanied by physiological arousal and expressive behaviors. Emotions can range from basic responses (such as fear or joy) to more complex states (like jealousy or guilt), influencing subjective experiences and behavior.

Cognition: Cognition encompasses mental processes involved in acquiring, understanding, and processing information. It includes perception, attention, memory, reasoning, problem-solving, and decision-making abilities.

2. Interdependence and Influence:

Biological Basis: Emotion and cognition are rooted in overlapping neural networks and physiological systems. The limbic system, including the amygdala and prefrontal cortex, plays a crucial role in integrating emotional responses with cognitive functions.

Mutual Influence: Emotions can shape cognitive processes by directing attention, influencing memory consolidation, and biasing decision-making. Similarly, cognitive appraisals and interpretations can modulate emotional responses, determining the intensity and duration of emotional experiences.

Mechanisms of Interaction
1. Attention and Perception:

Selective Attention: Emotional stimuli often capture attention more readily than neutral stimuli. This selective attention ensures prioritization of potentially significant information for survival and adaptive behavior.
Perceptual Bias: Emotions can influence perceptual processes, altering how individuals interpret and attribute meaning to sensory information. For instance, a person in a fearful state may perceive ambiguous stimuli as threatening.
2. Memory and Learning:

Emotional Memory: Emotionally salient events are often remembered more vividly and with greater detail compared to neutral events. This emotional enhancement of memory serves adaptive functions by facilitating learning from past experiences.

Learning and Conditioning: Emotional responses can facilitate learning and memory consolidation through processes such as classical and operant conditioning, where emotional associations influence behavioral responses.

3. Decision-Making and Problem-Solving:

Risk Assessment: Emotional states can bias decision-making processes by influencing perceptions of risk and reward. For example, heightened anxiety may lead to risk aversion, whereas positive emotions might promote risk-taking behaviors.

Problem-Solving Strategies: Emotions can foster creativity and innovative problem-solving strategies by encouraging divergent thinking and considering alternative perspectives beyond analytical approaches.

Practical Implications

1. Psychological Interventions:

Cognitive-Behavioral Therapy (CBT): Therapeutic approaches like CBT integrate cognitive restructuring and emotion regulation techniques to alleviate mood disorders and dysfunctional thinking patterns.

Mindfulness-Based Interventions: Practices promoting mindfulness enhance awareness of emotional and cognitive processes, fostering emotional regulation and adaptive coping strategies.

2. Education and Development:

Emotional Intelligence (EI): Educational programs emphasize EI competencies to promote self-awareness, empathy, and effective interpersonal skills among students, enhancing social-emotional learning and academic achievement.
3. Workplace Dynamics:

Leadership and Decision-Making: Effective leaders integrate emotional intelligence with cognitive abilities to navigate complex organizational challenges, foster team collaboration, and inspire employee engagement.
Conclusion
The interplay between emotion and cognition underscores their inseparable nature in shaping human behavior, perception, and interpersonal interactions. Understanding this dynamic relationship is essential for fostering emotional intelligence, promoting adaptive coping strategies, and optimizing cognitive functioning across diverse contexts. Continued research into the mechanisms and integration of emotion-cognition interactions contributes to advancing therapeutic interventions, educational practices, and organizational strategies aimed at enhancing individual well-being and collective success.

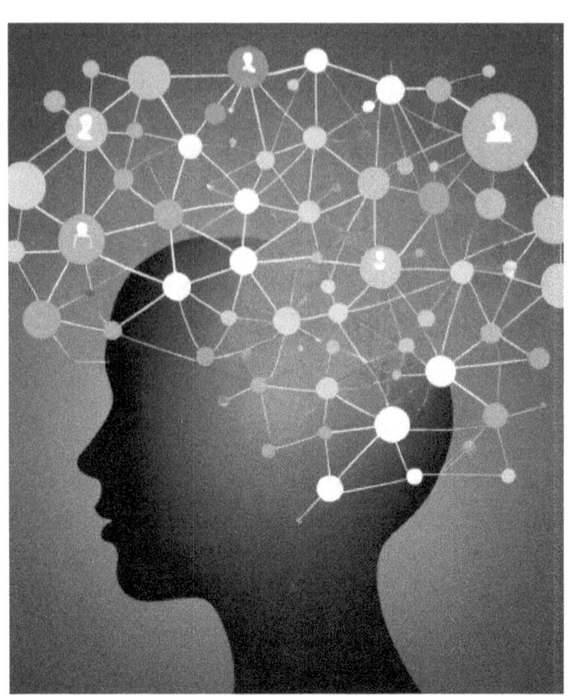

Chapter 24: The Art of Communication: Understanding Its Components

1. Verbal Communication:

Definition: Verbal communication involves the use of spoken or written words to convey messages. It includes language structure, vocabulary choice, and clarity of expression.
Importance: Clear and articulate verbal communication facilitates mutual understanding, exchange of information, and effective collaboration in interpersonal, professional, and social contexts.
Strategies: Enhancing verbal communication involves active listening, using appropriate tone and pitch, structuring coherent messages, and adapting language to the audience's comprehension level.
2. Nonverbal Communication:

Definition: Nonverbal communication encompasses gestures, facial expressions, body language, posture, eye contact, and other nonverbal cues that convey meaning and emotions.
Importance: Nonverbal cues often complement verbal messages, providing additional context, emotional expression, and sincerity in communication.
Strategies: Improving nonverbal communication skills involves maintaining eye contact, using open and confident body language, aligning gestures with verbal content, and interpreting nonverbal cues from others accurately.
3. Active Listening:

Definition: Active listening involves fully concentrating, understanding, responding, and remembering what is being communicated verbally and nonverbally.

Importance: Effective listening fosters empathy, builds trust, and enhances interpersonal relationships by demonstrating respect and genuine interest in others' perspectives.

Strategies: Practicing active listening includes paraphrasing, asking clarifying questions, reflecting emotions, and providing feedback to confirm understanding and validate speakers' experiences.

Barriers to Effective Communication

1. Communication Barriers:

Physical Barriers: Environmental factors such as noise, distance, and physical obstructions that hinder clear communication.

Psychological Barriers: Emotional states, biases, preconceptions, and cultural differences that affect interpretation and reception of messages.

Language Barriers: Differences in language proficiency, vocabulary, dialects, and communication styles that impede mutual comprehension.

2. Overcoming Communication Barriers:

Clear and Concise Messaging: Using simple language, avoiding jargon, and structuring messages logically to enhance clarity and comprehension.

Active Engagement: Encouraging feedback, verifying understanding, and adapting communication approaches to accommodate diverse audiences.

Cultural Sensitivity: Recognizing cultural norms, values, and communication customs to promote respectful and inclusive interactions.

Enhancing Communication Skills

1. Empathy and Emotional Intelligence:

Empathy: Understanding and sharing others' feelings, perspectives, and experiences to foster connection and mutual understanding.

Emotional Intelligence (EI): Managing emotions effectively, recognizing emotional cues in oneself and others, and adjusting communication styles accordingly.

2. Assertiveness and Conflict Resolution:

Assertiveness: Expressing thoughts, opinions, and needs confidently and respectfully, while considering others' viewpoints and maintaining interpersonal harmony.

Conflict Resolution: Using effective communication techniques to address disagreements, negotiate compromises, and achieve mutually beneficial outcomes.

Applications Across Contexts

1. Personal Relationships:

Building Trust: Establishing open and honest communication fosters trust, intimacy, and emotional support in familial, romantic, and platonic relationships.

Resolving Conflicts: Using active listening, empathy, and assertiveness to navigate conflicts and strengthen relationship bonds.

2. Professional Environments:

Leadership and Management: Effective communication skills are essential for leaders to articulate vision, inspire teams, delegate tasks, and foster a positive work culture.

Collaboration and Teamwork: Clear communication promotes collaboration, enhances productivity, and ensures alignment of goals and expectations among team members.

Conclusion

The art of communication encompasses verbal and nonverbal expressions, active listening, empathy, and strategies for overcoming barriers to effective communication. Developing and refining communication skills enhances interpersonal relationships, facilitates professional success, and contributes to personal growth by promoting clarity, understanding, and meaningful connections in diverse social and organizational contexts. Continual practice, self-awareness, and adaptation to varying communication needs and situations are key to mastering the art of communication in both personal and professional life.

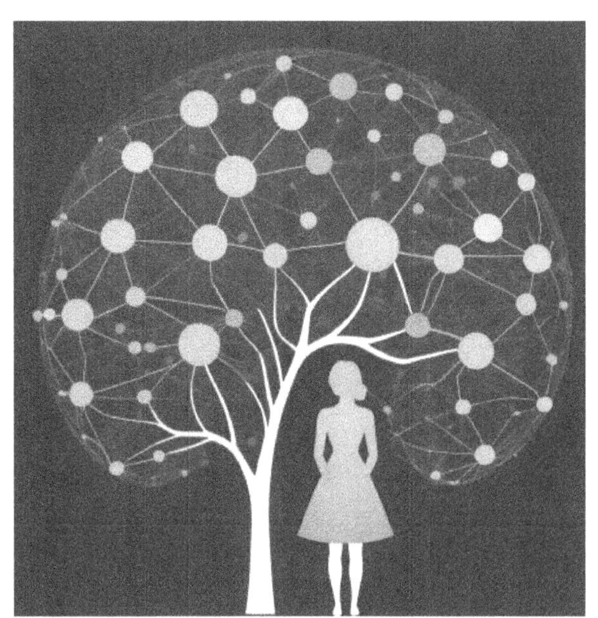

Chapter 25: Verbal Communication

Definition and Components:
Verbal communication involves the use of spoken or written words to convey messages. It includes:

Language Structure: The grammatical rules and syntax governing how words are organized into meaningful sentences.
Vocabulary Choice: The selection of words and phrases to accurately express ideas, emotions, and intentions.
Clarity of Expression: The ability to articulate thoughts in a coherent and understandable manner.
Importance:

Clarity and Precision: Verbal communication allows for precise expression of ideas and information, facilitating mutual understanding.
Information Exchange: It serves as a primary means for sharing knowledge, instructions, opinions, and feelings.
Social Function: Verbal communication enables storytelling, persuasion, negotiation, and social bonding.
Strategies for Effective Verbal Communication:

Active Listening: Paying attention to the speaker, asking clarifying questions, and providing feedback to ensure comprehension.
Clear and Concise Messaging: Avoiding ambiguity, using simple language, and structuring messages logically.
Adaptation to Audience: Adjusting language and tone based on the listener's familiarity with the topic and cultural context.
Nonverbal Communication

Definition and Components:
Nonverbal communication encompasses:

Gestures: Hand movements, facial expressions, and body posture that convey emotions and emphasis.
Facial Expressions: Visual cues involving the muscles of the face to display happiness, sadness, surprise, etc.
Body Language: Posture, stance, and physical movements that complement or contradict verbal messages.
Eye Contact: The duration and intensity of gaze, signaling interest, honesty, or authority.
Importance:

Emotional Expression: Nonverbal cues provide insights into a person's emotional state, authenticity, and sincerity.
Contextual Understanding: They add context and nuance to verbal messages, enhancing comprehension and empathy.
Relationship Building: Effective use of nonverbal cues fosters trust, rapport, and connection in interpersonal interactions.
Strategies for Effective Nonverbal Communication:

Awareness of Body Language: Monitoring posture, gestures, and facial expressions to align with verbal messages.
Regulating Emotions: Managing nonverbal cues to convey calmness, confidence, and approachability.
Interpreting Nonverbal Cues: Recognizing and responding to others' body language to gauge their emotional state and level of engagement.
Integration and Impact
Complementary Roles: Verbal and nonverbal communication often work together:

Consistency: When verbal and nonverbal cues align, messages are reinforced, enhancing clarity and credibility.

Contradiction: Inconsistencies can lead to confusion or misunderstanding, highlighting the importance of congruence in communication.
Adapting to Contexts: Effective communicators adjust their verbal and nonverbal behaviors based on:

Cultural Norms: Sensitivity to cultural differences in gestures, personal space, and eye contact.
Professional Settings: Tailoring communication styles for presentations, negotiations, interviews, and collaborative projects.
Conclusion
Mastering verbal and nonverbal communication involves awareness, practice, and adaptability across diverse interpersonal and professional contexts. By honing these skills, individuals can enhance their ability to convey ideas effectively, build meaningful relationships, and navigate complex social interactions with confidence and clarity.

Chapter 26: Barriers to Effective Communication

1. Physical Barriers:

Definition: Physical barriers hinder communication by obstructing the transmission or reception of messages.
Examples: Environmental noise, distance between communicators, poor lighting, and physical obstructions (e.g., walls) that limit visibility or auditory clarity.
Impact: Physical barriers can lead to misunderstandings, missed information, and reduced engagement in communication efforts.
2. Psychological Barriers:

Definition: Psychological factors influence how individuals perceive, interpret, and respond to communication.
Examples: Emotional states (e.g., stress, anxiety), biases, preconceptions, and mental health conditions that affect concentration or receptivity.
Impact: Psychological barriers may distort message reception, hinder active listening, and lead to misinterpretations or defensive responses.
3. Language Barriers:

Definition: Language barriers arise from differences in language proficiency, vocabulary, dialects, and communication styles.

Examples: Limited fluency in a shared language, technical jargon, cultural idioms, and nuances in meaning that vary across languages.

Impact: Language barriers can hinder comprehension, lead to misunderstandings, and limit effective communication across multicultural or multilingual settings.

4. Cultural Barriers:

Definition: Cultural barriers stem from differences in values, norms, beliefs, and communication customs between individuals or groups.

Examples: Nonverbal gestures (e.g., hand gestures, eye contact), personal space expectations, and culturally specific communication styles (e.g., direct vs. indirect communication).

Impact: Cultural barriers may lead to misinterpretations, offense, or alienation if communication norms and expectations are not understood or respected.

5. Technological Barriers:

Definition: Technological barriers pertain to issues related to the use of communication technology or tools.

Examples: Connectivity issues, malfunctioning equipment (e.g., microphone, video conferencing software), and unfamiliarity with digital communication platforms.

Impact: Technological barriers can disrupt communication flow, delay responses, and reduce the effectiveness of virtual or remote interactions.

Overcoming Communication Barriers

1. Clear and Concise Messaging:

Strategies: Using simple language, avoiding jargon, and structuring messages logically to enhance clarity and comprehension.

2. Active Engagement:

Strategies: Encouraging feedback, verifying understanding, and adapting communication approaches to accommodate diverse audiences.

3. Cultural Sensitivity:

Strategies: Recognizing cultural norms, values, and communication customs to promote respectful and inclusive interactions.

4. Technological Proficiency:

Strategies: Familiarizing oneself with communication tools, troubleshooting technical issues promptly, and practicing digital etiquette in virtual environments.

Conclusion

Identifying and addressing barriers to effective communication is essential for enhancing interpersonal relationships, teamwork, and organizational productivity. By recognizing and overcoming physical, psychological, language, cultural, and technological barriers, individuals and teams can foster clearer, more inclusive communication that promotes understanding, collaboration, and mutual respect across diverse contexts.

Chapter 27: Understanding Communication Skills

Definition: Communication skills encompass the abilities to convey thoughts, ideas, and information clearly and effectively to others. These skills are essential for expressing oneself, understanding others, and building rapport in various interpersonal and professional contexts.

Key Components of Communication Skills
1. Verbal Communication:

Definition: The use of spoken words to convey messages, ideas, and information.
Skills Involved: Clear articulation, vocabulary selection, tone modulation, and structured delivery.
Enhancement Strategies: Practice active listening, use concise language, and adapt communication style to the audience's understanding and preferences.
2. Nonverbal Communication:

Definition: Communication through body language, facial expressions, gestures, and eye contact.
Skills Involved: Interpreting and using nonverbal cues effectively to reinforce verbal messages, convey emotions, and gauge audience reactions.

Enhancement Strategies: Maintain eye contact, use open body posture, and align nonverbal cues with verbal communication to enhance clarity and authenticity.

3. Listening Skills:

Definition: The ability to actively receive, interpret, and respond to verbal and nonverbal messages from others.
Skills Involved: Paying attention, clarifying understanding, and empathizing with the speaker's perspective.
Enhancement Strategies: Practice active listening techniques such as paraphrasing, summarizing, and asking clarifying questions to demonstrate engagement and understanding.

4. Written Communication:

Definition: The ability to convey ideas, information, and messages through written words.
Skills Involved: Clarity, organization, grammar, and appropriate tone for the audience and purpose.
Enhancement Strategies: Proofreading, editing for clarity and conciseness, and adapting writing style to suit different formats (e.g., emails, reports, presentations).

5. Interpersonal Skills:

Definition: The ability to build and maintain relationships through effective communication, empathy, and respect.
Skills Involved: Conflict resolution, negotiation, empathy, and building rapport.
Enhancement Strategies: Develop empathy, practice assertiveness, and cultivate emotional intelligence to foster positive interactions and collaborative relationships.

Strategies for Enhancing Communication Skills

1. Practice Active Listening:

Engage fully in conversations, focus on the speaker's message, and avoid interrupting.

Reflect back what you hear to ensure understanding and show empathy.
2. Develop Clarity and Conciseness:

Use simple and precise language to convey ideas effectively.
Structure messages logically with clear main points and supporting details.
3. Seek and Provide Constructive Feedback:

Solicit feedback on your communication style and effectiveness.
Offer feedback to others tactfully to help them improve their communication skills.
4. Adapt Communication to Audience and Context:

Tailor your message based on the audience's knowledge, interests, and preferences.
Consider the cultural and situational context to ensure messages are relevant and respectful.
5. Continuously Learn and Improve:

Stay updated on communication trends, techniques, and best practices.
Seek opportunities for professional development, such as workshops, courses, or coaching, to refine your communication skills.
Benefits of Enhanced Communication Skills
Improved Relationships: Strengthen connections with colleagues, clients, friends, and family through clearer and more empathetic communication.
Increased Influence: Effectively convey ideas, persuade others, and inspire action through compelling communication.
Enhanced Career Success: Advance professionally by demonstrating strong communication abilities crucial for leadership, teamwork, and client interactions.
Conclusion

Enhancing communication skills involves developing proficiency in verbal and nonverbal communication, active listening, interpersonal interactions, and written communication. By continually refining these skills and adapting them to various contexts, individuals can build stronger relationships, achieve greater influence, and advance their personal and professional goals effectively.

Chapter 28: Self-Esteem

Definition: Self-esteem refers to an individual's overall subjective evaluation of their own worth and value. It encompasses feelings of self-respect, self-acceptance, and self-confidence.

Key Aspects of Self-Esteem:

Self-Worth: The belief in one's inherent value as a person, independent of external achievements or validation.

Self-Respect: Treating oneself with kindness, compassion, and dignity.

Self-Confidence: Trusting in one's abilities and judgment to navigate challenges and pursue goals.

Factors Influencing Self-Esteem:

Early Experiences: Childhood experiences, parenting styles, and interactions with caregivers shape early self-perceptions.

Social Comparisons: Comparing oneself to others can impact self-esteem, either positively or negatively, depending on perceived similarities or differences.

Achievements and Failures: Successes and setbacks in various domains (academic, professional, personal) can influence self-esteem.

Impact of High vs. Low Self-Esteem:

High Self-Esteem: Individuals with high self-esteem tend to be more resilient in the face of adversity, assertive in pursuing goals, and capable of forming healthy relationships.

Low Self-Esteem: Low self-esteem can contribute to feelings of inadequacy, self-doubt, and difficulty coping with challenges.

Self-Concept
Definition: Self-concept refers to the cognitive and evaluative perceptions an individual holds about themselves. It includes beliefs about personal characteristics, abilities, roles, and identities.

Components of Self-Concept:

Self-Identity: The sense of who one is, including roles (e.g., student, friend), attributes (e.g., intelligent, compassionate), and values.

Self-Image: How individuals perceive their physical appearance, strengths, weaknesses, and personality traits.

Ideal Self vs. Real Self: Discrepancies between one's perceived self (real self) and desired self (ideal self) can influence self-concept.

Formation and Development of Self-Concept:

Social Interactions: Feedback from others, social comparisons, and peer relationships contribute to shaping self-concept.

Cultural Influences: Cultural norms, values, and expectations shape self-concept by influencing identity development and self-perception.

Personal Experiences: Life experiences, achievements, failures, and challenges contribute to self-concept development over time.

Significance of Self-Esteem and Self-Concept:

Personal Well-Being: Positive self-esteem and a healthy self-concept contribute to emotional resilience, psychological health, and overall well-being.

Behavioral Outcomes: Individuals with positive self-esteem and a balanced self-concept are more likely to engage in adaptive behaviors, set realistic goals, and maintain motivation.

Enhancing Self-Esteem and Self-Concept
Self-Awareness: Reflect on strengths, weaknesses, values, and personal goals to gain clarity and understanding of oneself.

Positive Affirmations: Practice affirming positive qualities and achievements to reinforce self-esteem.

Set Realistic Goals: Break down larger goals into smaller, achievable steps to build a sense of accomplishment and self-efficacy.

Seek Support: Build a supportive network of friends, family, or mentors who provide encouragement and constructive feedback.

Challenge Negative Self-Talk: Identify and challenge self-critical thoughts or beliefs that undermine self-esteem and self-concept.

Conclusion
Self-esteem and self-concept are foundational aspects of individual identity and psychological well-being. By cultivating positive self-perceptions, setting realistic goals, and nurturing supportive relationships, individuals can enhance their self-esteem and develop a balanced self-concept that promotes resilience, personal growth, and overall life satisfaction.

Chapter 29: Developmental Stages of Self-Esteem

1. Early Childhood (Infancy to Age 5):

Foundation Building: Self-esteem begins to form as infants and young children develop a sense of trust and security through responsive caregiving.

Exploration and Mastery: Children build self-esteem through exploration, play, and learning new skills. Positive reinforcement and encouragement from caregivers play a crucial role in shaping early self-perceptions.

2. Middle Childhood (Ages 6 to 12):

Social Comparison: Children start comparing themselves to peers in terms of abilities, appearance, and social acceptance, influencing their self-esteem.

Competence and Achievement: Self-esteem is bolstered by successful experiences in school, sports, and hobbies. Academic performance and social acceptance become significant factors.

3. Adolescence (Ages 13 to 19):

Identity Formation: Adolescents navigate identity development, exploring personal values, beliefs, and roles. Self-esteem can fluctuate based on how well they perceive themselves fitting societal norms and expectations.

Peer Influence: Social acceptance and peer relationships play a pivotal role in shaping adolescents' self-esteem. Peer feedback, both positive and negative, can significantly impact self-perceptions.

4. Adulthood (Beyond Age 20):

Consolidation and Stability: Adults typically have a more stable sense of self-esteem based on accumulated life experiences, achievements, and relationships.

Life Transitions: Self-esteem may fluctuate during major life transitions such as career changes, relationships, and parenthood, depending on perceived success or challenges faced.

Factors Influencing Self-Esteem Development
1. Parental Influence:

Parenting Styles: Supportive, authoritative parenting fosters higher self-esteem, whereas authoritarian or neglectful parenting can hinder its development.

Attachment: Secure attachment in infancy lays a foundation for healthy self-esteem, fostering a sense of trust and competence.

2. Social Environment:

Peer Relationships: Acceptance by peers and positive social interactions contribute to higher self-esteem, while rejection or bullying can undermine it.

Cultural and Societal Influences: Cultural norms, societal expectations, and media portrayals influence self-esteem by shaping ideals of beauty, success, and achievement.

3. Personal Experiences:

Achievements and Failures: Successes and setbacks in academics, careers, relationships, and personal goals impact self-esteem.

Self-Perception: How individuals interpret and attribute meaning to their experiences affects their self-esteem. Positive self-talk and realistic self-appraisal can enhance self-esteem.

Enhancing and Maintaining Healthy Self-Esteem
1. Self-Awareness and Reflection:

Identify Strengths and Areas for Growth: Reflect on personal qualities, achievements, and areas needing improvement to build a balanced self-concept.
2. Positive Affirmations and Self-Compassion:

Celebrate Achievements: Acknowledge and celebrate successes, no matter how small, to reinforce positive self-perceptions.
3. Setting Realistic Goals:

Achievable Milestones: Break down larger goals into smaller, manageable steps to build confidence and a sense of accomplishment.
4. Seeking Support:

Social Network: Cultivate supportive relationships with friends, family, or mentors who provide encouragement and constructive feedback.

Conclusion

Self-esteem development is a lifelong process influenced by early experiences, social interactions, personal achievements, and cultural contexts. By fostering a supportive environment, promoting self-awareness, and cultivating resilience, individuals can enhance their self-esteem and cultivate a positive self-concept that supports their well-being and personal growth.

Chapter 30: Factors Affecting Self-Esteem

1. Early Experiences and Attachment:
Parental Relationships: The quality of attachment formed with caregivers during infancy and early childhood significantly influences self-esteem. Secure attachments foster feelings of trust, competence, and self-worth, while insecure attachments may lead to self-doubt and insecurity.

Parenting Styles: Supportive, authoritative parenting that balances warmth and discipline tends to promote higher self-esteem. In contrast, authoritarian or neglectful parenting styles can undermine self-esteem by either imposing unrealistic expectations or failing to provide adequate support and validation.

2. Social Relationships and Peer Influence:
Peer Acceptance: Acceptance and positive relationships with peers during childhood and adolescence are crucial for developing healthy self-esteem. Rejection or bullying can have detrimental effects on self-perception and confidence.

Social Comparisons: Individuals compare themselves to others to assess their own abilities, appearance, and achievements. Positive social comparisons can boost self-esteem, while negative comparisons may lead to feelings of inadequacy.

3. Cultural and Societal Influences:
Media and Society: Cultural ideals of beauty, success, and achievement portrayed in media can significantly impact self-esteem. Unrealistic standards and stereotypes can create pressure to conform and negatively influence self-perception.

Gender Roles: Societal expectations based on gender can shape self-esteem. For example, traditional gender norms may influence individuals' beliefs about their capabilities and roles, impacting their self-esteem accordingly.

4. Personal Experiences and Achievements:
Academic and Career Success: Achievements in academics, careers, and personal goals contribute to a sense of competence and accomplishment, boosting self-esteem. Conversely, repeated failures or setbacks can lower self-esteem if individuals perceive themselves as unsuccessful.

Life Transitions: Major life events such as starting a new job, ending a relationship, or facing health challenges can impact self-esteem. Successfully navigating transitions can enhance self-esteem by reinforcing resilience and adaptive coping skills.

5. Internal Factors and Self-Perception:
Self-Concept: How individuals perceive themselves, including their strengths, weaknesses, and overall self-image, influences self-esteem. Positive self-concept fosters higher self-esteem, while negative self-perceptions can undermine it.

Attribution Style: The way individuals attribute success or failure affects self-esteem. Those with an internal locus of control (believing they have control over outcomes) tend to have higher self-esteem compared to those with an external locus (attributing outcomes to external factors).

6. Psychological and Emotional Factors:
Emotional Regulation: Ability to manage and regulate emotions affects self-esteem. Poor emotional regulation skills may lead to self-criticism or feelings of inadequacy, while effective emotional management promotes a positive self-view.

Personality Traits: Traits such as resilience, optimism, and self-efficacy contribute to higher self-esteem by fostering adaptive coping strategies and a sense of personal competence.

7. Environmental and Socioeconomic Factors:
Family Environment: Socioeconomic status, family dynamics, and cultural background influence self-esteem. Supportive family environments and access to resources can enhance self-esteem, whereas economic hardships or familial conflicts may detract from it.

Educational and Community Support: Access to education, community support networks, and opportunities for skill development can positively impact self-esteem by providing avenues for personal growth and achievement.

Conclusion
Self-esteem is shaped by a complex interplay of early experiences, social interactions, cultural influences, personal achievements, and internal perceptions. Recognizing and understanding these factors can help individuals and practitioners develop strategies to enhance self-esteem, promote resilience, and foster a positive sense of self-worth across the lifespan.

Chapter 31: Strategies to Enhance Self-Esteem

1. Self-Awareness and Reflection
Identify Strengths and Weaknesses: Regular self-assessment helps individuals recognize their strengths and areas for improvement. This balanced view promotes self-acceptance and provides a foundation for growth.

Reflect on Achievements: Keeping a journal to document accomplishments, no matter how small, reinforces a positive self-image and reminds individuals of their capabilities.

2. Positive Self-Talk and Cognitive Restructuring
Challenge Negative Thoughts: Identify and question negative self-beliefs. Replace them with positive affirmations and realistic appraisals of situations.

Reframe Failures as Learning Opportunities: Viewing setbacks as opportunities for growth rather than as reflections of self-worth can transform how individuals perceive their capabilities.

3. Setting Realistic and Achievable Goals
Short-Term Goals: Break down larger objectives into smaller, manageable steps. Achieving these smaller goals provides a sense of accomplishment and boosts confidence.

Long-Term Vision: Having a clear long-term vision helps individuals stay focused and motivated, providing direction and purpose.

4. Building Competence and Mastery
Skill Development: Engage in activities that enhance skills and knowledge. Mastery of new abilities builds competence and self-esteem.

Continuous Learning: Embrace lifelong learning. Pursuing new interests and hobbies can enhance self-esteem by broadening one's capabilities and knowledge base.

5. Social Support and Positive Relationships
Surround Yourself with Positive People: Build a support network of friends, family, and mentors who provide encouragement and constructive feedback.

Seek Support When Needed: Don't hesitate to seek help from mental health professionals or support groups when facing challenges. Professional guidance can provide valuable insights and coping strategies.

6. Healthy Lifestyle Choices
Physical Health: Regular exercise, a balanced diet, and adequate sleep contribute to overall well-being and a positive self-image.

Mental Health: Engage in activities that promote mental health, such as mindfulness, meditation, or relaxation techniques. A healthy mind supports positive self-esteem.

7. Emotional Regulation and Resilience
Emotional Awareness: Recognize and understand your emotions. Being aware of emotional triggers and responses can help manage reactions and maintain self-esteem.

Develop Resilience: Cultivate resilience by practicing coping strategies that help you bounce back from adversity. This includes maintaining a positive outlook and learning from challenges.

8. Practicing Self-Compassion
Be Kind to Yourself: Treat yourself with the same kindness and understanding you would offer to a friend. Acknowledge mistakes without harsh self-criticism.

Forgive Yourself: Let go of past mistakes and forgive yourself. Holding on to guilt or regret can undermine self-esteem.

9. Engagement in Meaningful Activities
Volunteering and Altruism: Helping others and engaging in community service can enhance self-esteem by fostering a sense of purpose and connectedness.

Pursue Passions: Engage in activities that you are passionate about. Passion-driven pursuits often lead to personal fulfillment and enhanced self-esteem.

10. Assertiveness Training
Communicate Your Needs: Learn to express your needs, desires, and opinions confidently and respectfully. Assertiveness fosters a sense of control and self-respect.

Set Boundaries: Establish and maintain healthy boundaries in relationships. Respecting your own limits and ensuring others do the same is crucial for self-esteem.

Conclusion

Enhancing self-esteem is a multifaceted process that involves cognitive, emotional, and behavioral strategies. By fostering self-awareness, practicing positive self-talk, setting realistic goals, building competence, and maintaining supportive relationships, individuals can develop a healthy and resilient sense of self-worth. These strategies not only promote self-esteem but also contribute to overall well-being and life satisfaction.

Chapter 32: Group Dynamics and Social Influence

Group dynamics and social influence are critical areas of study in social psychology, as they explain how individuals behave, think, and feel within a group setting. Understanding these concepts is essential for recognizing the impact groups have on personal behavior and societal norms.

Group Dynamics
Definition and Importance:
Group dynamics refers to the interactions and processes that occur between members of a group. These interactions shape the group's structure, cohesion, and performance. Understanding group dynamics is vital for improving teamwork, communication, and productivity in various settings, such as workplaces, schools, and social organizations.

Key Concepts:

Group Formation and Development:

Stages of Group Development: Groups typically go through stages such as forming, storming, norming, performing, and adjourning. Each stage represents different levels of group interaction, conflict resolution, and goal achievement.
Group Cohesion: Cohesion refers to the bonds that hold the group together. High cohesion usually leads to better communication and collaboration but can also result in groupthink, where the desire for harmony suppresses dissenting opinions.
Roles and Norms:

Roles: Roles are the expected behaviors assigned to individuals within the group. They can be formal (e.g., a team leader) or informal (e.g., a peacemaker). Clear roles help in organizing tasks and responsibilities.
Norms: Norms are the unwritten rules and expectations for behavior within the group. They guide interactions and ensure conformity, promoting group stability and functioning.
Leadership:

Types of Leadership: Different leadership styles (e.g., autocratic, democratic, laissez-faire) impact group dynamics. Effective leaders can motivate and guide their groups towards achieving goals while maintaining morale and cohesion.
Influence of Leadership: Leaders play a crucial role in shaping group norms, resolving conflicts, and making decisions that affect group performance and satisfaction.
Communication Patterns:

Formal and Informal Communication: Effective communication within a group can be formal (structured, official) or informal (casual, spontaneous). Both types are essential for sharing information, building relationships, and coordinating efforts.

Barriers to Communication: Miscommunication, lack of clarity, and cultural differences can hinder group functioning. Overcoming these barriers is critical for maintaining effective group dynamics.

Social Influence

Definition and Importance:

Social influence refers to the ways in which individuals change their behavior to meet the demands of a social environment. It encompasses the processes through which individuals' thoughts, feelings, and actions are affected by others. Understanding social influence is crucial for recognizing how societal norms, peer pressure, and authority impact personal and group behavior.

Key Concepts:

Conformity:

Types of Conformity: Conformity involves changing behavior to align with group norms. It can be informational (believing the group is correct) or normative (seeking social approval). Asch's Conformity Experiments: These classic experiments demonstrated the power of group pressure on individuals' willingness to conform, even when the group is clearly wrong.

Compliance:

Techniques of Compliance: Compliance refers to changing behavior in response to a direct request. Techniques such as the foot-in-the-door (starting with a small request) and door-in-the-face (starting with a large request) can increase compliance rates. Factors Influencing Compliance: Factors like authority, social proof, and scarcity can significantly affect individuals' willingness to comply with requests.

Obedience:

Milgram's Obedience Study: This landmark study highlighted the extent to which individuals would obey authority figures, even to the point of causing harm to others. It underscored the power of authority in shaping behavior.

Ethical Considerations: The study raised important ethical questions about the treatment of participants and the potential for abuse of authority.

Group Polarization:

Definition: Group polarization occurs when group discussions lead to more extreme positions than initially held by individual members. This can result in heightened risk-taking or stronger convictions.

Mechanisms: Mechanisms such as social comparison (aligning with perceived group norms) and persuasive arguments (being swayed by dominant viewpoints) contribute to polarization.

Groupthink:

Symptoms and Consequences: Groupthink is a phenomenon where the desire for consensus in decision-making leads to poor judgments and overlooked alternatives. Symptoms include an illusion of invulnerability, collective rationalization, and suppression of dissenting opinions.

Prevention: Encouraging open dialogue, seeking external opinions, and fostering a culture of critical evaluation can help prevent groupthink.

Conclusion

Understanding group dynamics and social influence provides valuable insights into how individuals interact within groups and how group settings can shape behaviors, attitudes, and decisions. By recognizing the underlying principles and factors that drive group interactions and social influence, individuals and organizations can enhance collaboration, improve decision-making processes, and foster healthier, more productive social environments.

Chapter 33: Formation and Functioning of Groups

The formation and functioning of groups are central to understanding social behavior and interactions. Groups influence individuals' thoughts, actions, and feelings, making the study of their formation and functioning essential for various fields such as psychology, sociology, organizational behavior, and education.

Formation of Groups
Stages of Group Development:

Forming:

Initial Stage: During this stage, individuals come together and begin to understand the group's purpose. Members are usually polite, cautious, and trying to figure out their place within the group.

Characteristics: Uncertainty, excitement, anxiety, and guarded interactions. There is a focus on orientation and getting acquainted.
Storming:

Conflict Emergence: As members become more comfortable, conflicts may arise due to differing opinions, personalities, and working styles.
Characteristics: Disagreements, competition, and tension. This stage is crucial for the growth of the group as it addresses power struggles and clarifies roles.
Norming:

Developing Cohesion: The group starts to establish norms, roles, and stronger relationships. Members begin to trust each other and work more harmoniously.
Characteristics: Cooperation, consensus, and team cohesion. The group sets clear goals and develops a shared sense of purpose.
Performing:

Efficient Functioning: The group reaches a stage where it functions effectively towards achieving its goals. Roles are clear, and processes are streamlined.
Characteristics: High productivity, strong cooperation, and problem-solving. The group can handle complex tasks and conflicts constructively.
Adjourning:

Disbanding: This final stage occurs when the group has accomplished its goals and begins to disband.
Characteristics: Reflection, celebration of achievements, and planning for the future. Members may feel a sense of loss or accomplishment.
Functioning of Groups
Group Structure:

Roles:

Defined Roles: Specific responsibilities and expectations assigned to each member, which help in organizing tasks and reducing ambiguity.
Role Clarity: Clear understanding of individual roles enhances efficiency and reduces conflicts. Role ambiguity can lead to stress and dissatisfaction.
Norms:

Unwritten Rules: Norms are the informal rules that govern behavior within the group. They develop organically and guide interactions.
Establishment: Norms are established through interactions and experiences. They can promote stability and predictability but may also stifle creativity if too rigid.
Status:

Hierarchical Position: Status refers to the relative social position or rank of group members. It influences interactions, influence, and decision-making.
Impact on Behavior: Higher status individuals often have more influence and control over group processes. Status differences can create power dynamics that affect group cohesion.
Group Cohesion:

Attraction to the Group:

Interpersonal Attraction: Cohesion increases when members are attracted to each other and the group's goals. Positive relationships enhance commitment and satisfaction.
Task Cohesion: Focus on achieving common goals and objectives strengthens group unity.
Cohesiveness Factors:

Similarity: Shared interests, values, and backgrounds enhance cohesion.
Size: Smaller groups tend to be more cohesive due to easier communication and stronger bonds.
Success: Achieving goals together boosts morale and cohesion.
Communication Patterns:

Formal Communication:

Structured Interactions: Formal communication follows established channels and procedures, such as meetings, reports, and official memos. It ensures clarity and accountability.
Importance: It is essential for coordinating tasks, disseminating information, and making decisions.
Informal Communication:

Casual Interactions: Informal communication includes spontaneous and casual interactions, such as water-cooler conversations and social gatherings.
Role: It builds relationships, fosters trust, and can lead to creative problem-solving. Informal networks often facilitate quicker information flow.
Decision-Making Processes:

Consensus:

Group Agreement: Reaching a decision that all members can support. It fosters buy-in and commitment but can be time-consuming.
Process: Involves discussion, negotiation, and compromise to reach a mutually acceptable solution.
Majority Rule:

Voting: Decisions are made based on the preference of the majority. It is efficient but may lead to dissatisfaction among the minority.
Implementation: Common in democratic groups and organizations. It requires clear procedures for voting and decision enforcement.
Authority Rule:

Leader Decision: A designated leader or authority figure makes the decision, sometimes with input from the group. It is quick but may not always consider all perspectives.
Effectiveness: Best suited for situations requiring swift action or when expertise is concentrated in one individual.
Conflict Resolution:

Types of Conflict:

Task Conflict: Disagreements about the content and goals of the work. Can be constructive if managed well.
Relationship Conflict: Personal incompatibilities and emotional tensions. Often destructive and needs careful management.
Process Conflict: Disagreements about how tasks should be accomplished. Can be disruptive but also an opportunity for improvement.
Conflict Management Strategies:

Avoidance: Ignoring the conflict. Suitable for minor issues but can lead to unresolved tension.
Accommodation: Yielding to others' needs. Maintains harmony but may lead to resentment.
Competition: Asserting one's viewpoint at the expense of others. Effective for decisive action but can harm relationships.
Compromise: Each party gives up something. Resolves conflicts quickly but may result in suboptimal solutions.

Collaboration: Working together to find a win-win solution.
Ideal for achieving the best outcome but requires time and
effort.
Conclusion
Understanding the formation and functioning of groups is
crucial for fostering effective and harmonious group
interactions. By recognizing the stages of group development,
the structural elements that influence group behavior, and the
dynamics of communication, decision-making, and conflict
resolution, individuals and organizations can enhance group
performance, satisfaction, and overall success.

Chapter 34: Roles and Norms Within Groups

Roles and norms are foundational elements of group
dynamics that significantly influence how groups function
and achieve their objectives. Understanding these concepts is
crucial for anyone involved in group settings, whether in
professional, academic, or social contexts. Here is an in-depth
exploration of roles and norms within groups:

Roles Within Groups
Definition of Roles:

Roles are defined positions within a group that outline specific
behaviors, responsibilities, and expectations assigned to
individual members. Each role serves a particular function
that contributes to the group's overall objectives.
Types of Roles:

Task Roles:

Definition: These roles focus on the accomplishment of group objectives and tasks.
Examples:
Initiator/Contributor: Proposes new ideas and approaches.
Information Seeker: Requests clarification and information.
Coordinator: Organizes and integrates group activities.
Evaluator: Critically assesses the group's progress and outcomes.
Maintenance Roles:

Definition: These roles aim to maintain positive relationships and group cohesion.
Examples:
Encourager: Provides support and encouragement to others.
Harmonizer: Mediates conflicts and reduces tension.
Gatekeeper: Facilitates participation from all members.
Follower: Supports group decisions and helps implement plans.
Individual Roles:

Definition: These roles are often self-centered and may detract from group goals.
Examples:
Aggressor: Criticizes or deflates others to assert dominance.
Blocker: Opposes ideas and resists progress without offering alternatives.
Recognition Seeker: Seeks attention through personal achievements.
Dominator: Tries to control the group's direction and decisions.
Role Clarity and Ambiguity:

Role Clarity:

Definition: When group members clearly understand their own roles and the roles of others, it leads to better coordination and reduced conflict.
Benefits: Enhanced performance, increased satisfaction, and effective task completion.
Strategies for Clarity: Providing detailed role descriptions, setting clear expectations, and offering regular feedback.
Role Ambiguity:

Definition: Uncertainty about one's role, responsibilities, or expectations.
Consequences: Increased stress, reduced motivation, and potential conflicts.
Mitigation: Regular communication, role negotiation, and adjustment of responsibilities as needed.
Role Conflict:

Definition:

Occurs when there are incompatible demands placed upon an individual by two or more roles, or when the expectations of different roles clash.
Types:

Inter-role Conflict: Conflict between roles in different groups (e.g., work and family roles).
Intra-role Conflict: Conflict within a single role due to competing demands.
Resolution:

Prioritizing roles, seeking support from group members, and negotiating role expectations can help resolve conflicts.
Norms Within Groups
Definition of Norms:

Norms are the informal, often unspoken, rules that govern the behavior of group members. They are established through group interactions and shared experiences.
Characteristics of Norms:

Implicit vs. Explicit:

Implicit Norms: Unwritten and understood through social cues and behaviors.
Explicit Norms: Clearly stated and formally documented, often through group agreements or codes of conduct.
Descriptive vs. Injunctive:

Descriptive Norms: Describe how members typically behave.
Injunctive Norms: Describe how members should behave according to the group's values and expectations.
Functions of Norms:

Regulating Behavior:

Norms help standardize behavior within the group, ensuring predictability and order.
Facilitating Group Survival:

By promoting behaviors that support group objectives and cohesion, norms enhance the group's ability to function effectively.
Defining Social Reality:

Norms shape perceptions and interpretations of acceptable behavior, influencing the group's culture and identity.
Expressing Group Values:

Norms reflect the underlying values and beliefs of the group, reinforcing a shared sense of identity and purpose.
Formation and Enforcement of Norms:

Formation:

Norms develop organically as group members interact, share experiences, and respond to specific situations. They can also be established intentionally through discussion and agreement.
Enforcement:

Compliance: Members conform to norms to gain acceptance and avoid conflict.
Sanctions: Positive reinforcement (rewards) for adherence and negative consequences (punishments) for violations.
Changing Norms:

Recognition:

Acknowledging that existing norms may no longer be effective or relevant.
Process:

Discussing the need for change, involving all members in the decision-making process, and gradually introducing new norms.
Resistance:

Anticipating and addressing resistance to change through clear communication, education, and demonstrating the benefits of new norms.
Conclusion

Roles and norms are integral to the effective functioning of groups. Roles define the structure and responsibilities within the group, ensuring tasks are accomplished and relationships are maintained. Norms provide a framework for acceptable behavior, promoting group cohesion and efficiency. Understanding and managing roles and norms are essential for achieving group objectives and fostering a positive group environment.

Chapter 35: Influence of Group Behavior on Individuals

Group behavior significantly impacts individual behavior, shaping attitudes, actions, and perceptions. Understanding these influences is crucial for anyone involved in group dynamics, whether in professional, educational, or social settings. Here is an in-depth exploration of how group behavior affects individuals:

Social Influence
Definition:

Social influence refers to the ways in which individuals change their behavior to meet the demands of a social environment. This influence can be direct or indirect and is a fundamental aspect of group dynamics.
Types of Social Influence:

Conformity:

Definition: The tendency to align one's attitudes, beliefs, and behaviors with those of a group.
Examples: Changing personal opinions to match the majority view, adopting group norms in dress or speech.
Factors Influencing Conformity:
Group Size: Larger groups often exert more pressure to conform.
Unanimity: The presence of a unanimous group opinion increases conformity.
Cohesion: Higher group cohesion leads to greater conformity.
Compliance:

Definition: Adapting behavior in response to a direct request from another person or group.
Examples: Following instructions from a team leader, participating in group activities even if reluctant.
Techniques for Compliance:
Foot-in-the-Door: Starting with a small request to increase the likelihood of agreement to a larger request.
Door-in-the-Face: Making a large request expecting refusal, followed by a smaller, more reasonable request.
Obedience:

Definition: Following orders or instructions from an authority figure.

Examples: Employees following directives from their manager, soldiers following commands from their superiors.
Factors Influencing Obedience:
Authority: The perceived legitimacy and expertise of the authority figure.
Responsibility: Belief that the authority figure is responsible for the outcomes.
Proximity: Closer physical or psychological proximity to the authority figure increases obedience.
Group Dynamics and Individual Behavior
Group Polarization:

Definition: The tendency for group discussions to lead to decisions that are more extreme than the initial inclinations of the group members.
Examples: Political discussions leading to more extreme political views, business meetings resulting in riskier or more conservative decisions than initially proposed.
Mechanisms:
Informational Influence: Exposure to additional arguments reinforcing the initial viewpoint.
Normative Influence: Desire to be accepted and liked by group members, leading to stronger expressions of the prevailing opinion.
Groupthink:

Definition: A mode of thinking that people engage in when they are deeply involved in a cohesive group, where the desire for unanimity overrides the motivation to appraise alternative courses of action.
Examples: Historical decisions such as the Bay of Pigs invasion, business blunders due to lack of critical evaluation.
Symptoms:
Illusion of Invulnerability: Overconfidence in the group's decisions.

Collective Rationalization: Discounting warnings and negative feedback.
Self-Censorship: Withholding dissenting views to maintain harmony.
Prevention:
Encouraging Open Debate: Promoting a culture where dissent is valued.
Assigning a Devil's Advocate: Designating someone to question assumptions and decisions.
Breaking into Smaller Groups: Ensuring diverse perspectives are considered.
Social Facilitation:

Definition: The tendency for people to perform better on simple tasks in the presence of others, but worse on complex tasks.
Examples: Athletes performing better in front of a crowd, students solving easier problems faster when observed but struggling with difficult problems.
Explanation:
Arousal: Presence of others increases physiological arousal, enhancing performance on well-learned tasks but impairing performance on tasks requiring complex or new skills.
Social Loafing:

Definition: The tendency for individuals to put in less effort when working in a group compared to when working alone.
Examples: Group projects where some members contribute less, teams where a few members carry the workload.
Factors Reducing Social Loafing:
Individual Accountability: Ensuring each member's contributions are identifiable.
Task Importance: Emphasizing the significance of each member's role.
Group Cohesion: Fostering a sense of belonging and commitment to the group's goals.

Interpersonal Relationships in Groups
Interpersonal Attraction:

Definition: The degree to which individuals are drawn to each other within the group.
Factors Influencing Attraction:
Similarity: Shared interests, values, and backgrounds.
Proximity: Physical closeness and frequent interactions.
Reciprocal Liking: Mutual positive feelings and support.
Conflict and Cooperation:

Conflict:
Definition: Disagreement and discord arising from differences in ideas, interests, or values.
Types: Task conflict (disagreements about the content of tasks) and relationship conflict (personal incompatibilities).
Resolution: Open communication, negotiation, and mediation.
Cooperation:
Definition: Working together towards common goals.
Promoting Cooperation: Establishing shared goals, building trust, and fostering interdependence.
Conclusion
Understanding the influence of group behavior on individuals is essential for effectively navigating and managing group dynamics. Social influences such as conformity, compliance, and obedience shape individual behavior, while group phenomena like polarization and groupthink impact decision-making processes. Recognizing and addressing these influences can enhance group performance, foster positive interactions, and mitigate potential conflicts, ultimately leading to more successful and harmonious group outcomes.

Chapter 36: The Power of Persuasion

Persuasion is a fundamental aspect of human interaction, influencing attitudes, beliefs, and behaviors. Understanding the principles and techniques of persuasion can be invaluable in various fields, including marketing

The Power of Persuasion

Persuasion is a fundamental aspect of human interaction, influencing attitudes, beliefs, and behaviors. Understanding the principles and techniques of persuasion is invaluable in various fields, including marketing, politics, law, and everyday social interactions. This chapter explores the principles of persuasion, the techniques and strategies used, and the ethical considerations involved.

Principles of Persuasion
Reciprocity

Definition: People tend to return favors. If someone does something for us, we feel obligated to repay them.
Examples: Free samples in a store encourage purchases, charitable organizations sending small gifts to potential donors.
Applications: Use this principle to build goodwill by offering something valuable upfront, creating a sense of obligation.
Commitment and Consistency

Definition: Once people commit to something, they are more likely to follow through to remain consistent with their initial commitment.
Examples: Signing a petition increases the likelihood of later voting on the issue, initial small commitments leading to larger ones (foot-in-the-door technique).
Applications: Start with small requests to gain commitment, which can be leveraged for larger actions later.
Social Proof

Definition: People look to others to determine their own behavior, especially in uncertain situations.
Examples: Testimonials, user reviews, and displaying customer numbers or social media followers.
Applications: Highlight popularity or approval from others to encourage similar behavior from new individuals.

Authority

Definition: People tend to obey figures of authority or those perceived as experts.
Examples: Doctors endorsing health products, experts giving opinions on media.
Applications: Use endorsements from credible experts or authorities in the relevant field to build trust and persuade.
Liking

Definition: People are more easily persuaded by others they like.
Examples: Celebrity endorsements, attractive and personable salespeople.
Applications: Build rapport and connect personally with the audience to increase persuasive effectiveness.
Scarcity

Definition: Limited availability increases the perceived value and desire for an item.
Examples: Limited-time offers, limited edition products, highlighting unique features.
Applications: Create a sense of urgency or exclusivity to motivate quick decisions.
Techniques and Strategies
Foot-in-the-Door Technique

Description: Start with a small request to gain compliance, then follow with a larger request.
Example: Asking someone to sign a petition and later asking for a donation.
Effectiveness: Works because initial small commitments lead to a desire to be consistent with subsequent actions.
Door-in-the-Face Technique

Description: Make a large request expecting it to be refused, then follow up with a smaller, more reasonable request.
Example: Asking for a large donation and then a smaller one.
Effectiveness: The smaller request seems more reasonable in comparison to the larger one, and people feel a sense of obligation to reciprocate the perceived concession.
Low-Balling

Description: Get someone to commit to a lower-cost request and then raise the stakes.
Example: Car sales where a lower price is initially offered, then additional fees are added.
Effectiveness: Once committed, people are likely to follow through despite increased costs.
That's-Not-All Technique

Description: Offer something additional to make the deal more appealing before the person can respond.
Example: "But wait, there's more!" offers in infomercials.
Effectiveness: Perceived additional value enhances the attractiveness of the offer.
Framing

Description: Present information in a way that influences perception and decision-making.
Example: Describing a glass as "half full" instead of "half empty."
Effectiveness: Positive or negative framing can significantly affect attitudes and choices.
Ethical Considerations in Persuasion
Honesty and Transparency

Description: Being truthful and clear about intentions and outcomes.
Importance: Builds trust and long-term credibility.

Risks: Misleading or deceptive practices can lead to loss of trust and legal consequences.
Respecting Autonomy

Description: Allowing individuals to make their own decisions without undue pressure or manipulation.
Importance: Preserves the dignity and freedom of choice.
Risks: Coercion or manipulation undermines autonomy and can lead to ethical breaches.
Avoiding Exploitation

Description: Not taking advantage of individuals' vulnerabilities or lack of knowledge.
Importance: Ensures fairness and respect in interactions.
Risks: Exploitative practices can cause harm and damage reputations.
Informed Consent

Description: Ensuring that individuals understand what they are agreeing to and the implications.
Importance: Upholds ethical standards and legal requirements.
Risks: Failure to obtain informed consent can result in ethical violations and legal repercussions.
Conclusion
Persuasion is a powerful tool that, when used ethically, can positively influence attitudes and behaviors. By understanding the principles of reciprocity, commitment, social proof, authority, liking, and scarcity, and employing techniques such as foot-in-the-door, door-in-the-face, low-balling, and framing, one can effectively persuade others while maintaining ethical integrity. Recognizing the responsibility that comes with the power of persuasion is crucial for fostering trust, respect, and positive social interactions.

Chapter 37: Principles of Persuasion

Understanding the principles of persuasion is essential for effectively influencing others. These principles are rooted in psychological research and demonstrate consistent patterns in human behavior. Below are the six key principles of persuasion:

1. Reciprocity
Definition: The principle of reciprocity states that people feel obligated to return favors or kindnesses. When someone does something for us, we naturally want to repay them.

Examples:

Marketing: Free samples or trial periods. When consumers receive something for free, they are more likely to purchase the product.
Social Interactions: Inviting a friend to a party makes them more likely to invite you to their events.
Applications:

Business: Offering complimentary services or gifts can foster goodwill and encourage customers to reciprocate with purchases or referrals.
Personal Relationships: Small acts of kindness can strengthen bonds and create a cycle of positive exchanges.
2. Commitment and Consistency
Definition: People prefer to be consistent with their commitments. Once they have made a choice or taken a stand, they are more likely to behave consistently with that commitment.

Examples:

Public Declarations: Asking people to make public commitments increases the likelihood they will follow through (e.g., signing a pledge to donate to a cause).
Foot-in-the-Door Technique: Getting someone to agree to a small request increases the chances they will agree to a larger request later.
Applications:

Marketing: Encouraging customers to start with a small purchase or trial can lead to more substantial future commitments.
Personal Development: Setting small, achievable goals helps build a pattern of success and consistency.
3. Social Proof
Definition: People look to others to guide their own behavior, especially in uncertain situations. This principle asserts that we determine what is correct by finding out what other people think is correct.

Examples:

Online Reviews: Positive reviews and ratings from other users influence potential buyers.
Behavioral Cues: In a restaurant, if everyone is ordering a particular dish, newcomers are more likely to choose the same.
Applications:

Marketing: Highlighting testimonials and customer feedback can increase credibility and attract new customers.
Event Planning: Promoting popular events with high attendance numbers can encourage more people to attend.
4. Authority
Definition: People tend to follow the lead of credible, knowledgeable experts. Authority figures have a significant influence on behavior and decisions.

Examples:

Expert Endorsements: Doctors endorsing health products or celebrities recommending a brand.
Uniforms and Titles: Police officers, doctors, and other professionals in uniform or with recognized titles command respect and compliance.

Applications:

Marketing: Using endorsements from industry experts or influencers can enhance the perceived value of a product.
Leadership: Demonstrating expertise and knowledge can help leaders gain trust and motivate their teams.
5. Liking
Definition: People are more easily persuaded by others they like. Factors such as physical attractiveness, similarity, compliments, and cooperative efforts can enhance liking.

Examples:

Sales Techniques: Salespeople building rapport with customers by finding common ground or offering genuine compliments.
Social Media Influencers: Followers are more likely to trust and be influenced by influencers they find relatable and likable.
Applications:

Customer Relations: Building genuine relationships and finding commonalities with clients can improve sales and loyalty.
Networking: Developing a friendly and approachable demeanor can facilitate better connections and collaborations.
6. Scarcity
Definition: Perceived scarcity generates demand. When something is in limited supply, people perceive it as more valuable and are more likely to want it.

Examples:

Limited-Time Offers: Promotions with deadlines, such as "Only 24 hours left!" or "Limited stock available."

Exclusive Products: Items marketed as exclusive or limited edition increase their desirability.
Applications:

Sales: Creating a sense of urgency or exclusivity can drive quick decisions and increase sales.
Event Planning: Promoting limited tickets or seats can enhance interest and prompt faster registrations.
Conclusion
The principles of persuasion—reciprocity, commitment and consistency, social proof, authority, liking, and scarcity—provide a robust framework for influencing others effectively and ethically. Understanding these principles allows individuals and organizations to create strategies that foster positive and lasting impacts. Whether in marketing, leadership, or everyday interactions, these principles help in crafting persuasive messages and actions that resonate with people on a fundamental psychological level.

Chapter 38: Techniques and Strategies of Persuasion

Understanding the principles of persuasion is foundational, but applying them effectively requires specific techniques and strategies. Below are key techniques and strategies that leverage the principles of persuasion to influence behavior and decision-making:

1. Foot-in-the-Door Technique
Definition: This technique involves getting a person to agree
to a small request as a way of increasing the likelihood that
they will agree to a larger request later.

Example: A charity might ask you to sign a petition (a small
request) and then later ask for a donation (a larger request).

Strategy:

Initial Engagement: Start with an easy, non-threatening
request to build initial agreement.
Gradual Escalation: Once initial compliance is achieved,
gradually increase the magnitude of requests.
Application:

Sales: Get customers to try a free sample or a low-cost trial,
making them more likely to purchase the full product later.
Activism: Gain support through small actions like signing up
for a newsletter, then escalate to larger commitments like
attending events or making donations.
2. Door-in-the-Face Technique
Definition: This technique involves making a large request
that is expected to be refused, followed by a smaller, more
reasonable request.

Example: Asking someone to donate $500 to a cause (likely to
be refused) and then asking for a smaller $50 donation (more
likely to be accepted).

Strategy:

Initial Overreach: Present an unreasonably large request that
is likely to be declined.

Concession: Follow up with a significantly smaller request, creating a sense of obligation to reciprocate the concession.
Application:

Fundraising: Start with a high donation request to make subsequent smaller amounts seem more reasonable.
Negotiation: Begin negotiations with high demands, then make concessions that lead to mutually acceptable agreements.
3. Anchoring
Definition: This cognitive bias involves using an initial piece of information (the anchor) to influence subsequent judgments and decisions.

Example: Setting a high initial price for a product and then offering a discount to make the sale price seem more attractive.

Strategy:

Initial Anchor: Provide an initial reference point that sets the stage for further discussion.
Comparative Value: Highlight how subsequent options compare favorably to the initial anchor.
Application:

Pricing: Introduce a high-end model first, making mid-range models seem more affordable by comparison.
Negotiations: Start with an ambitious opening offer to influence the perception of reasonable counteroffers.
4. Social Proof
Definition: Leveraging the behavior of others to influence individuals, based on the idea that people tend to follow the actions of the majority.

Example: Displaying customer testimonials and reviews on a website to build trust and credibility.

Strategy:

Visibility: Make positive behaviors and endorsements visible and prominent.
Relevance: Use examples and testimonials from peers or relatable individuals.
Application:

Marketing: Use user-generated content, reviews, and testimonials to demonstrate widespread approval and satisfaction.
Events: Highlight the number of attendees or participants to encourage more people to join.
5. Scarcity
Definition: Creating a perception of limited availability to increase demand.

Example: Promoting a product as a "limited edition" or offering a "limited-time sale."

Strategy:

Urgency: Use time-sensitive language to create a sense of urgency (e.g., "Offer ends soon").
Exclusivity: Emphasize the rarity or unique aspects of the offering.
Application:

Sales: Run flash sales or limited-time offers to drive immediate purchases.
Memberships: Offer exclusive access or early-bird specials to create a sense of privilege.
6. Authority

Definition: Using the endorsement or approval of experts and authority figures to lend credibility.

Example: Featuring a well-known doctor in an advertisement for a health product.

Strategy:

Credible Endorsements: Utilize endorsements from recognized experts or authorities in the field.
Visible Credentials: Highlight qualifications, certifications, or awards.
Application:

Advertising: Use expert testimonials and industry certifications to enhance product credibility.
Content: Publish white papers or case studies authored by reputable figures.
7. Reciprocity
Definition: Leveraging the human tendency to return favors and acts of kindness.

Example: Sending a free gift to potential customers to increase the likelihood they will make a purchase.

Strategy:

Initial Giving: Provide value upfront through free samples, valuable content, or small gifts.
Follow-up: Make subsequent requests that feel like a natural reciprocation.
Application:

Customer Loyalty: Offer free trials or gifts to create a sense of obligation to continue the relationship.

Networking: Offer help or resources first to build reciprocal professional relationships.
8. Liking
Definition: People are more likely to be persuaded by those they like and find attractive.

Example: Building rapport and finding common ground with a potential client before making a pitch.

Strategy:

Build Rapport: Engage in genuine conversation and find common interests.
Positive Interaction: Use compliments and cooperative behavior to build a positive relationship.
Application:

Sales: Develop personal connections with clients to build trust and likability.
Team Building: Foster a positive, friendly work environment to enhance cooperation and productivity.
Conclusion
These techniques and strategies of persuasion, grounded in psychological principles, can be powerful tools when used ethically and responsibly. Whether in marketing, sales, negotiation, or everyday interactions, understanding how to apply these methods can enhance one's ability to influence and motivate others effectively. By leveraging techniques such as the foot-in-the-door, door-in-the-face, anchoring, social proof, scarcity, authority, reciprocity, and liking, individuals can craft persuasive messages and actions that resonate and lead to desired outcomes.

Chapter 39: Ethical Considerations in Persuasion

Persuasion is a powerful tool that can influence attitudes, beliefs, and behaviors. However, its potency also comes with significant ethical responsibilities. Ethical considerations in persuasion ensure that this influence is wielded responsibly, respecting the autonomy and dignity of individuals. Here are the key ethical considerations to keep in mind:

1. Respect for Autonomy

Definition: This principle involves acknowledging and respecting the decision-making rights of others.

Details:

Informed Consent: Ensure that the audience is fully informed about the nature and purpose of the persuasive attempt.
Transparency: Avoid deceptive practices. Be honest about intentions, benefits, and potential drawbacks.
Application:

Marketing: Provide clear, truthful information about products or services without exaggeration or omission of critical details.
Healthcare: Ensure patients are fully informed about treatment options and their implications before making decisions.
2. Non-Coercion
Definition: Ethical persuasion avoids using force, manipulation, or undue pressure to achieve compliance.

Details:

Voluntary Acceptance: Persuasion should allow for free and voluntary acceptance or rejection of the message.
Avoiding Manipulation: Refrain from exploiting psychological vulnerabilities or emotional states.
Application:

Sales: Ensure that sales tactics do not rely on high-pressure techniques or emotional manipulation.
Negotiations: Engage in fair and balanced discussions, allowing all parties to consent freely to terms.
3. Truthfulness and Accuracy
Definition: Presenting information truthfully and accurately is foundational to ethical persuasion.

Details:

Fact-Checking: Verify all claims and data before presenting them.
Honesty: Avoid misleading statistics, selective omission of facts, or false endorsements.
Application:

Advertising: Ensure that advertisements are truthful and not misleading or exaggerated.
Political Campaigns: Promote honest discourse, fact-check statements, and avoid spreading misinformation.
4. Beneficence and Non-Maleficence
Definition: These principles involve promoting good and preventing harm through persuasive efforts.

Details:

Positive Impact: Ensure that the persuasive effort aims to benefit the audience or society at large.
Avoid Harm: Avoid messages or tactics that could cause physical, psychological, or social harm.
Application:

Public Health Campaigns: Design campaigns that encourage beneficial behaviors (e.g., vaccination) without causing undue fear or anxiety.
Corporate Responsibility: Avoid promoting harmful products or services, even if they are profitable.
5. Fairness and Justice
Definition: Ensuring that persuasive efforts are fair and just involves treating all individuals and groups equitably.

Details:

Equitable Treatment: Avoid discrimination or bias in persuasive messages.
Accessibility: Make information accessible to all, including marginalized or disadvantaged groups.
Application:

Education: Provide equal access to educational materials and opportunities for persuasion.
Public Policy: Ensure that policies and their promotion do not disproportionately benefit or harm specific groups.
6. Respect for Privacy
Definition: Respecting the privacy of individuals means not intruding into their personal lives without consent.

Details:

Data Protection: Ensure the confidentiality and security of any personal information gathered.
Consent: Obtain explicit consent before using personal information for persuasive purposes.
Application:

Digital Marketing: Adhere to data protection regulations and obtain consent for the use of personal data.
Research: Protect the privacy of research participants and use their data ethically.
Conclusion

Ethical persuasion is about balancing the power of influence with the responsibility of respect and integrity. Practitioners must commit to transparency, respect for autonomy, truthfulness, beneficence, fairness, and privacy. By adhering to these ethical principles, persuasive efforts can achieve their goals without compromising the well-being and rights of individuals and society. This approach not only fosters trust and credibility but also ensures that the influence exercised is just and constructive, contributing positively to the collective social fabric.

Chapter 40: The Role of Empathy in Social Connections

Empathy plays a critical role in forming and maintaining social connections. It enables individuals to understand and share the feelings of others, which fosters deeper and more meaningful relationships. Here, we explore the importance of empathy in various aspects of social interactions.

1. Understanding Empathy
Definition: Empathy is the ability to recognize, understand, and share the thoughts and feelings of another person. It involves both cognitive and emotional components.

Details:

Cognitive Empathy: This refers to the intellectual ability to understand someone else's perspective or mental state.
Emotional Empathy: This involves actually feeling the emotions that another person is experiencing.
Application:

Interpersonal Relationships: Empathy allows for better communication and connection by understanding and validating others' emotions and viewpoints.
Conflict Resolution: Empathy helps in de-escalating conflicts by allowing individuals to see the situation from the other party's perspective.
2. Empathy's Impact on Relationships
Definition: Empathy is essential for building trust, cooperation, and intimacy in relationships.

Details:

Trust Building: When people feel understood and validated, they are more likely to trust and open up to others.
Cooperation: Empathetic individuals are better at working together, as they can anticipate and respond to the needs and emotions of their peers.
Intimacy: Empathy enhances emotional closeness by facilitating deeper, more authentic connections.
Application:

Romantic Relationships: Empathy strengthens bonds by promoting understanding and support, crucial for emotional intimacy.
Friendships: Friends who empathize with each other are better at offering support and maintaining strong, lasting connections.
3. Cultivating Empathy
Definition: Empathy can be developed and enhanced through conscious effort and practice.

Details:

Active Listening: Fully focusing on the speaker, understanding their message, and responding thoughtfully.
Perspective-Taking: Deliberately trying to see things from another person's point of view.
Emotional Regulation: Managing one's own emotions to better understand and respond to others' emotions.
Application:

Training Programs: Empathy training for professionals in fields such as healthcare, education, and customer service to improve interpersonal skills.
Personal Practice: Mindfulness and reflective practices that enhance self-awareness and emotional intelligence.
4. Empathy in Professional Settings

Definition: Empathy is a valuable skill in the workplace, enhancing leadership, teamwork, and customer relations.

Details:

Leadership: Empathetic leaders are more effective, as they understand and address the needs and concerns of their team members.
Teamwork: Teams with empathetic members tend to have better communication, collaboration, and conflict resolution.
Customer Relations: Empathy improves customer service by ensuring that customers feel heard, understood, and valued.
Application:

Leadership Development: Incorporating empathy training into leadership programs to foster more supportive and effective leaders.
Customer Service Training: Teaching empathy as part of customer service protocols to enhance customer satisfaction and loyalty.
5. Empathy and Mental Health
Definition: Empathy has significant implications for mental health, both for individuals and communities.

Details:

Support Systems: Empathy is the foundation of effective support systems, providing emotional and psychological support to those in need.
Community Well-Being: Communities that cultivate empathy tend to be more inclusive, supportive, and resilient.
Application:

Counseling and Therapy: Empathy is crucial for therapists and counselors to build rapport and effectively support their clients.

Community Programs: Initiatives that promote empathy, such as anti-bullying campaigns and peer support groups, contribute to healthier, more supportive communities.
Conclusion
Empathy is a cornerstone of human social connections, enhancing understanding, trust, cooperation, and emotional closeness. It plays a vital role in personal relationships, professional settings, and community well-being. By cultivating empathy through active listening, perspective-taking, and emotional regulation, individuals and societies can build stronger, more supportive networks. Empathy not only enriches personal interactions but also contributes to the overall mental health and harmony of communities, making it an essential skill for both personal and social development.

Chapter 41: Understanding Empathy

Empathy is a complex psychological phenomenon essential for human interactions and social cohesion. It involves the ability to understand and share the feelings, thoughts, and perspectives of others. Here's a detailed exploration of empathy, including its components, development, and significance.

Components of Empathy
1. Cognitive Empathy:

Definition: Cognitive empathy refers to the intellectual ability to understand another person's perspective or mental state. Details: It involves accurately perceiving and comprehending the emotions, thoughts, and intentions of others through observation and inference.
Application: Cognitive empathy enables individuals to anticipate reactions, understand social norms, and navigate interpersonal relationships effectively.
2. Emotional Empathy:

Definition: Emotional empathy involves feeling the same or similar emotions as another person in response to their experiences.
Details: It is characterized by a visceral reaction to someone else's emotional state, leading to shared emotional experiences.
Application: Emotional empathy fosters compassion, support, and bonding in relationships by validating and resonating with others' feelings.
3. Compassionate Empathy:

Definition: Compassionate empathy combines cognitive understanding with a genuine concern for the well-being of others.

Details: It motivates individuals to take action to alleviate suffering or support others based on their understanding and emotional resonance.

Application: Compassionate empathy drives prosocial behavior, such as helping behaviors, altruism, and moral decision-making, contributing to a supportive and caring society.

Development of Empathy

1. Early Childhood:

Formation: Empathy begins to develop in infancy through caregivers' responsiveness to the child's emotional cues.

Progression: It evolves during childhood and adolescence through social interactions, role modeling, and emotional regulation.

Factors: Parental warmth, secure attachments, and exposure to diverse social experiences play crucial roles in empathy development.

2. Adulthood:

Continued Growth: Empathy continues to mature in adulthood through life experiences, cultural influences, and cognitive development.

Stress and Resilience: Challenges and adversity can either enhance empathy through shared experiences or diminish it through emotional fatigue and desensitization.

Training and Education: Empathy can be cultivated and enhanced through empathy training programs, mindfulness practices, and interpersonal skills development.

Significance of Empathy

1. Interpersonal Relationships:

Foundation: Empathy forms the basis of trust, intimacy, and emotional connection in personal relationships.

Conflict Resolution: It facilitates understanding and reconciliation by validating emotions and perspectives during conflicts.

Support Networks: Empathetic relationships provide emotional support, comfort, and encouragement during challenging times.

2. Professional Contexts:

Leadership: Empathetic leaders inspire trust, foster teamwork, and enhance employee well-being and productivity.

Customer Relations: Empathy improves customer satisfaction, loyalty, and retention by addressing needs and concerns effectively.

Healthcare: Empathy is crucial for patient-centered care, enhancing therapeutic relationships and treatment outcomes.

3. Societal Impact:

Social Cohesion: Empathy promotes tolerance, cooperation, and inclusivity, contributing to harmonious communities and societal well-being.

Global Perspective: Empathetic understanding of diverse cultures, beliefs, and experiences fosters cross-cultural understanding and peaceful coexistence.

Conclusion

Empathy is a multifaceted ability essential for navigating complex social interactions, fostering meaningful relationships, and promoting collective well-being. Understanding its cognitive, emotional, and compassionate dimensions allows individuals and societies to cultivate empathy effectively. By prioritizing empathy in personal interactions, professional settings, and societal initiatives, individuals can contribute to a more empathetic and compassionate world, where understanding and supporting others are fundamental values.

Chapter 42: Empathy's Impact on Relationships

Empathy plays a pivotal role in shaping the dynamics and quality of relationships across various contexts, from personal to professional settings. Here's an expert exploration of how empathy influences relationships and why it is crucial for interpersonal connection.

1. Foundation of Trust and Connection
Definition: Empathy involves understanding and sharing the emotions of others, which fosters mutual trust and emotional connection.
Details: When individuals feel understood and validated, they are more likely to build trust and openness in their relationships.
Application: Empathetic listening and responsiveness create a safe space for partners, friends, or colleagues to express themselves authentically without fear of judgment.
2. Enhanced Communication
Definition: Empathy improves communication by enabling individuals to perceive and interpret verbal and nonverbal cues accurately.
Details: Empathetic individuals are adept at active listening, clarifying emotions, and validating others' perspectives.
Application: Effective communication built on empathy strengthens relationships, resolves conflicts constructively, and enhances mutual understanding.
3. Support and Emotional Resonance
Definition: Empathy allows individuals to emotionally resonate with others' experiences and provide meaningful support.

Details: Empathetic responses validate emotions, offering comfort, reassurance, and encouragement during difficult times.

Application: Supportive relationships grounded in empathy promote emotional well-being, resilience, and a sense of belonging.

4. Conflict Resolution and Understanding

Definition: Empathy facilitates understanding of differing viewpoints and promotes empathy-driven conflict resolution.

Details: By acknowledging and validating diverse perspectives, empathetic individuals navigate conflicts with empathy and compassion.

Application: Resolving conflicts through empathetic dialogue fosters mutual respect, strengthens relationships, and prevents misunderstandings.

5. Intimacy and Bonding

Definition: Empathy deepens emotional intimacy by creating authentic connections and shared emotional experiences.

Details: Empathetic partners or friends connect on a deeper level, fostering intimacy, closeness, and emotional support.

Application: Strong emotional bonds nurtured by empathy promote relationship satisfaction, longevity, and resilience to challenges.

6. Mutual Growth and Support

Definition: Empathy promotes personal growth and mutual support by encouraging individuals to understand and respond to each other's needs.

Details: Empathetic relationships thrive on reciprocity, mutual care, and the willingness to support each other's growth and development.

Application: By fostering empathy, relationships become enriching partnerships where both parties feel valued, understood, and supported in achieving their goals.

Conclusion

Empathy serves as a cornerstone of healthy, fulfilling relationships by fostering trust, effective communication, emotional support, conflict resolution, intimacy, and mutual growth. Cultivating empathy allows individuals to build strong, resilient connections that enhance their overall well-being and contribute to a harmonious social environment. As such, prioritizing empathy in relationships—whether personal, professional, or communal—creates a foundation for empathy-driven interactions that promote understanding, compassion, and positive relational outcomes.

Chapter 43: Cultivating Empathy

Empathy, the ability to understand and share the feelings of others, is a skill that can be nurtured and developed over time through conscious effort and practice. Here's an expert exploration of how individuals can cultivate empathy in various aspects of their lives.

1. Active Listening
Definition: Active listening involves fully concentrating, understanding, responding to, and remembering what is being said.
Details: Empathetic listening requires paying attention to both verbal and nonverbal cues, such as tone of voice, facial expressions, and body language.
Application: Practice reflective listening by paraphrasing what the other person has said to demonstrate understanding and validate their feelings.
2. Perspective-Taking
Definition: Perspective-taking is the ability to see a situation from another person's point of view.
Details: Empathy involves stepping into someone else's shoes mentally and imagining their thoughts, emotions, and experiences.
Application: Engage in role-playing exercises or storytelling to practice understanding different perspectives and empathizing with diverse viewpoints.
3. Cultivating Curiosity
Definition: Cultivating curiosity involves maintaining an open mind and a genuine interest in understanding others.
Details: Ask open-ended questions to explore others' thoughts, feelings, and motivations without making assumptions or judgments.

Application: Practice curiosity in everyday interactions by seeking to learn about others' backgrounds, interests, and experiences.

4. Mindfulness Practices

Definition: Mindfulness involves being present in the moment with non-judgmental awareness of one's thoughts, feelings, and sensations.

Details: Mindfulness enhances empathy by increasing self-awareness and sensitivity to others' emotional cues.

Application: Incorporate mindfulness techniques such as deep breathing, meditation, or body scan exercises to develop emotional awareness and empathetic responses.

5. Cultural Competence

Definition: Cultural competence is the ability to understand, communicate with, and effectively interact with people across different cultures.

Details: Empathy extends to recognizing and respecting cultural differences in beliefs, values, and communication styles.

Application: Engage in cross-cultural experiences, learn about diverse cultural norms and practices, and actively seek to understand cultural contexts to enhance empathetic understanding.

6. Empathy-Building Activities

Definition: Empathy-building activities are structured exercises designed to enhance empathetic skills and promote understanding.

Details: Activities may include volunteer work, group discussions, role-playing scenarios, or participating in community events.

Application: Participate in empathy workshops or group activities that encourage perspective-taking, active listening, and collaborative problem-solving.

7. Self-Reflection and Feedback

Definition: Self-reflection involves introspection and examination of one's thoughts, feelings, and behaviors.

Details: Regular self-reflection allows individuals to assess their empathetic responses, identify areas for improvement, and learn from past interactions.

Application: Seek constructive feedback from trusted individuals to gain insights into how others perceive your empathetic abilities and adjust behavior accordingly.

Conclusion

Cultivating empathy involves developing a combination of skills, attitudes, and behaviors that foster understanding, compassion, and interpersonal connection. By actively practicing active listening, perspective-taking, curiosity, mindfulness, cultural competence, engaging in empathy-building activities, and engaging in self-reflection, individuals can strengthen their empathetic abilities and contribute to building more empathetic and supportive relationships, communities, and societies. Empathy is a fundamental aspect of emotional intelligence and plays a crucial role in promoting positive social interactions, resolving conflicts, and fostering mutual understanding and respect among diverse individuals and groups.

Chapter 44: Interpersonal Relationships and Social Cognition

Interpersonal relationships are fundamental to human interaction and are deeply intertwined with social cognition—the processes involved in perceiving, interpreting, and understanding others' thoughts, emotions, and behaviors. Here's an expert explanation of how social cognition influences interpersonal relationships:

1. Perception of Others
Definition: Social cognition begins with the perception of others, where individuals interpret cues such as facial expressions, body language, and verbal communication to form initial impressions.
Details: These perceptions are influenced by schemas, mental frameworks that organize and interpret information about people and social situations based on past experiences and cultural norms.
Application: Understanding how perceptions shape interactions helps individuals navigate relationships more effectively by recognizing biases and adjusting interpretations.
2. Attribution Theory
Definition: Attribution theory examines how individuals explain the causes of behavior, whether attributing it to internal factors (personality traits) or external factors (situational circumstances).
Details: Attributional biases, such as the fundamental attribution error (attributing others' behaviors to internal characteristics while overlooking situational factors), impact interpersonal judgments.

Application: Recognizing attributional biases promotes empathetic understanding by considering context and mitigating misunderstandings in relationships.

3. Social Cognitive Biases

Definition: Social cognitive biases are systematic errors in thinking that influence perceptions of others and decision-making in social contexts.

Details: Biases like confirmation bias (seeking information that confirms existing beliefs) or halo effect (generalizing one positive trait to overall perception) shape interpersonal interactions.

Application: Awareness of biases fosters critical thinking and reduces stereotyping, enhancing accurate perceptions and promoting more authentic relationships.

4. Theory of Mind

Definition: Theory of mind refers to the ability to attribute mental states — beliefs, intentions, desires — to oneself and others and understand that others have perspectives different from one's own.

Details: Developing theory of mind supports perspective-taking, empathy, and understanding diverse viewpoints essential for successful interpersonal relationships.

Application: Practicing theory of mind enhances communication, conflict resolution, and cooperation by acknowledging and respecting others' perspectives and emotions.

5. Social Cognitive Development

Definition: Social cognitive development refers to the lifelong process of acquiring social knowledge, skills, and abilities necessary for navigating complex social environments.

Details: From infancy to adulthood, individuals learn social norms, etiquettes, and relational dynamics through observation, imitation, and direct experience.

Application: Understanding social cognitive development informs strategies for building healthy relationships across different life stages and cultural contexts.

Conclusion
Interpersonal relationships are intricately linked to social cognition, encompassing how individuals perceive, interpret, and respond to others in social contexts. By understanding the principles of social cognition — perception, attribution theory, social cognitive biases, theory of mind, and social cognitive development — individuals can cultivate empathy, improve communication, resolve conflicts effectively, and build meaningful and supportive relationships. Enhancing social cognitive skills contributes to personal growth, promotes social harmony, and fosters mutual understanding and respect in diverse interpersonal interactions.

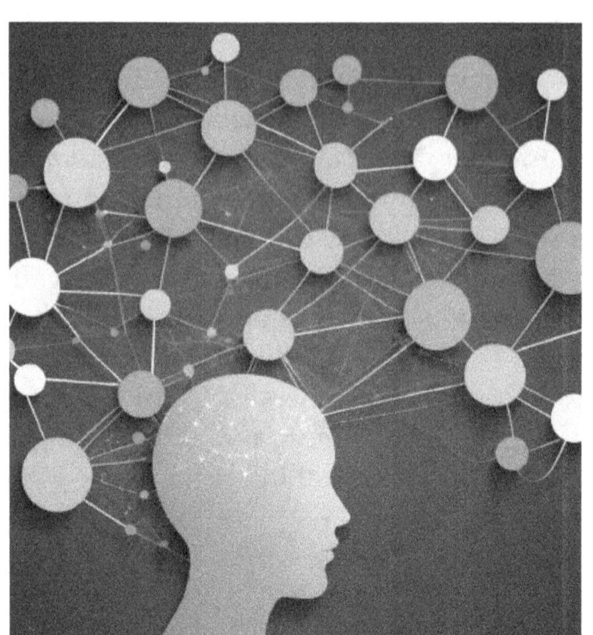

Chapter 45: How We Perceive and Think About Others

Understanding how individuals perceive and think about others is fundamental to navigating social interactions and building meaningful relationships. Here's an expert explanation of the processes involved:

1. Perception of Others
Definition: Perception involves interpreting sensory information (visual, auditory, tactile) to form impressions of others.
Details: Perception is influenced by physical appearance, body language, facial expressions, tone of voice, and contextual cues.
Application: Awareness of perceptual biases (e.g., stereotyping based on appearance) helps individuals engage in more accurate and empathetic interactions.
2. Schemas and Stereotypes
Definition: Schemas are mental frameworks that organize knowledge and expectations about people, situations, and social roles.
Details: Stereotypes are generalized beliefs about groups or categories of people based on perceived characteristics.
Application: Recognizing and challenging stereotypes promotes fair and equitable treatment, fostering inclusive and respectful interpersonal relationships.
3. Impression Formation
Definition: Impression formation refers to the process of developing initial perceptions and evaluations of others.
Details: Factors influencing impression formation include first impressions, central traits (prominent characteristics), and primacy and recency effects (early and recent information).

Application: Cultivating positive first impressions and considering multiple sources of information supports accurate and nuanced understanding of others.

4. Attribution Processes

Definition: Attribution involves explaining the causes of behavior — whether attributing it to internal factors (personality, abilities) or external factors (situations, environment).

Details: Attributional biases, such as the fundamental attribution error (overestimating internal factors and underestimating situational factors), influence judgments.

Application: Considering situational factors and context improves understanding and reduces misunderstandings in interpersonal interactions.

5. Social Identity Theory

Definition: Social identity theory posits that individuals define themselves in part by their group memberships and strive for positive social identity.

Details: Ingroup bias (favoring one's own group) and outgroup derogation (negative attitudes toward other groups) impact social perceptions.

Application: Promoting awareness of social identities and fostering intergroup empathy enhances cooperation and reduces prejudice in relationships.

6. Cognitive Biases

Definition: Cognitive biases are systematic patterns of deviation from rationality in judgment, affecting perceptions and decision-making.

Details: Biases like confirmation bias (seeking information confirming preexisting beliefs) or halo effect (generalizing one positive trait to overall judgment) shape perceptions.

Application: Critical thinking and mindfulness mitigate cognitive biases, fostering accurate and empathetic perceptions of others.

Conclusion

How individuals perceive and think about others is influenced by complex cognitive processes, including perception, schemas and stereotypes, impression formation, attribution processes, social identity theory, and cognitive biases. By understanding these mechanisms, individuals can cultivate empathy, improve interpersonal communication, challenge stereotypes, and promote positive social interactions. Developing awareness of perceptual biases and fostering inclusive attitudes enhances personal relationships, supports diversity, and contributes to building cohesive communities based on mutual respect and understanding.

Chapter 46: Attribution Theory

Attribution theory is a psychological framework that explores how individuals interpret the causes of behavior, both their own and others'. Developed by Fritz Heider in the 1950s and expanded upon by subsequent researchers such as Harold Kelley and Bernard Weiner, attribution theory seeks to explain the reasoning processes behind why people behave the way they do and how they attribute these behaviors to internal or external factors.

1. Internal vs. External Attribution
Definition: Attribution theory distinguishes between internal attributions (attributing behavior to personal traits, abilities, or dispositions) and external attributions (attributing behavior to situational factors or environmental influences).
Details: Internal attributions might include traits like intelligence or personality, while external attributions could involve factors such as luck or situational constraints.
Application: Understanding whether someone's behavior is due to their inherent qualities or the circumstances they are in helps individuals make sense of and predict others' actions.
2. Types of Attribution Biases
Fundamental Attribution Error: This bias refers to the tendency to overemphasize internal factors when explaining others' behavior while underestimating the impact of external factors. For example, attributing someone's tardiness to laziness rather than traffic.

Actor-Observer Bias: This bias occurs when explaining one's own behavior (actor) versus others' behavior (observer). Actors tend to attribute their actions to external factors (e.g., situational pressures), while observers attribute similar behaviors to internal factors (e.g., personality traits).

3. Attributional Dimensions
Stability: Stability refers to whether the cause of behavior is perceived as enduring or temporary. Stable attributions suggest consistency over time (e.g., intelligence), while unstable attributions imply variability (e.g., mood).

Controllability: Controllability relates to whether the cause of behavior is within the individual's control. Attributes like effort and skill are perceived as controllable, whereas factors like luck or natural ability may be seen as uncontrollable.

4. Applications in Everyday Life
Interpersonal Relationships: Attribution theory helps individuals understand conflicts or misunderstandings in relationships by considering whether behaviors are due to personal traits or external circumstances.

Education and Work: Teachers and managers can use attribution theory to provide feedback effectively. Praising effort (internal, controllable attribution) rather than intelligence (internal, stable attribution) promotes motivation and resilience.

5. Critiques and Limitations
Cultural Differences: Attributional tendencies may vary across cultures, influencing how behavior is interpreted and evaluated.

Complexity: Human behavior is often multifaceted, making it challenging to attribute solely to internal or external factors. Context and individual differences also play significant roles.

Conclusion

Attribution theory provides a framework for understanding the complex processes involved in how individuals perceive and explain behavior. By recognizing the biases and dimensions of attribution, individuals can enhance their interpersonal relationships, improve communication, and make more accurate judgments about others' actions. Moreover, applying attribution theory in various contexts — from personal interactions to educational and organizational settings — facilitates effective problem-solving, decision-making, and conflict resolution.

Chapter 47: Social Cognitive Biases

Social cognitive biases are systematic errors in thinking that influence how individuals perceive themselves, others, and the world around them. These biases can impact judgments, decisions, and interactions in various social contexts. Here's an expert explanation of some key social cognitive biases:

1. Confirmation Bias
Definition: Confirmation bias is the tendency to search for, interpret, favor, and recall information that confirms one's preexisting beliefs or hypotheses.
Details: People selectively gather evidence that supports their beliefs while ignoring or downplaying contradictory information.
Application: In social situations, confirmation bias can lead to misunderstandings, reinforce stereotypes, and hinder objective analysis of others' behaviors.
2. Halo Effect
Definition: The halo effect occurs when a person's overall impression of someone (based on one positive trait) influences their perceptions of other traits.
Details: For example, if someone is perceived as physically attractive, they might also be judged as intelligent or kind, even without direct evidence.
Application: The halo effect can impact hiring decisions, social interactions, and personal evaluations, potentially leading to biased judgments.
3. Stereotyping
Definition: Stereotyping involves categorizing individuals or groups based on perceived characteristics, traits, or behaviors.

Details: Stereotypes are generalized beliefs that may be based on race, gender, age, profession, or other attributes, and they often involve overgeneralization and oversimplification.
Application: Stereotypes can influence behavior, expectations, and interactions, leading to prejudice, discrimination, and unfair treatment.
4. Ingroup Bias
Definition: Ingroup bias is the tendency to favor members of one's own group (ingroup) over those who belong to other groups (outgroups).
Details: This bias can lead to loyalty, solidarity, and positive attitudes toward ingroup members, while outgroup members may be viewed more negatively or unfairly.
Application: Ingroup bias influences social identity, group dynamics, and intergroup relations, impacting social cohesion and intergroup conflicts.
5. Attributional Biases
Fundamental Attribution Error: As previously mentioned, this bias involves attributing others' behavior to internal factors (personality, disposition) rather than external factors (situational context).

Actor-Observer Bias: This bias refers to differences in attributions made for one's own behavior (actor attributing to external factors) versus others' behavior (observer attributing to internal factors).

6. False Consensus Effect
Definition: The false consensus effect is the tendency for people to overestimate the extent to which others share their beliefs, attitudes, and behaviors.
Details: Individuals may assume that their own opinions are more widespread or typical than they actually are, which can lead to miscommunication and misunderstanding.

Application: This bias affects decision-making, social influence, and the perception of social norms within a group or community.

Conclusion

Social cognitive biases are pervasive in human cognition and can significantly influence social perceptions, interactions, and judgments. By understanding these biases, individuals can become more aware of their own thought processes and mitigate their impact on interpersonal relationships, decision-making, and societal dynamics. Awareness and critical thinking skills are essential for recognizing and addressing biases, promoting empathy, fairness, and effective communication in diverse social contexts.

Chapter 48: The Influence of Social Norms

Social norms are societal expectations, rules, and guidelines that dictate appropriate behavior in various social contexts. These norms influence how individuals think, feel, and behave, shaping cultural practices, interpersonal relationships, and group dynamics. Here's an expert explanation of the influence of social norms:

1. Definition and Types of Social Norms
Definition: Social norms are implicit or explicit rules that govern acceptable behavior within a particular group, community, or society.
Types:
Descriptive Norms: These norms define what behaviors are typically performed in a given situation. For example, standing in line at a store or speaking softly in a library.
Injunctive Norms: These norms specify what behaviors are approved or disapproved by others. They represent social approval or disapproval of certain actions.
2. How Norms Shape Behavior
Social Control: Norms act as a form of social control, guiding individuals towards conformity and discouraging deviant behavior.
Normative Influence: Individuals conform to norms to gain social acceptance, avoid rejection, or maintain social harmony.

Internalization: Over time, norms become internalized as personal beliefs and values, influencing self-regulation and decision-making.

3. Changing and Challenging Norms

Social Change: Norms evolve over time in response to societal shifts, cultural movements, and demographic changes.

Deviance and Innovation: Challenging norms can lead to social change and innovation, but it may also provoke resistance or social sanctions.

Cultural Variability: Norms vary across cultures and subcultures, reflecting diverse values, traditions, and social expectations.

4. Examples of Social Norms

Gender Norms: Expectations regarding behaviors, roles, and characteristics deemed appropriate for men and women.

Etiquette Norms: Guidelines for polite and respectful behavior in social interactions, such as table manners or greetings.

Legal Norms: Laws and regulations that govern acceptable conduct and define consequences for violations.

5. Impact on Behavior and Decision-Making

Conformity: Individuals conform to norms to fit in, avoid conflict, or gain social approval, even if it contradicts personal beliefs.

Normative Social Influence: The desire to conform to group norms influences behavior in public settings, such as conformity experiments like Asch's line experiment.

Identity and Self-Expression: Norms shape identity formation and influence how individuals express themselves within social contexts.

6. Ethical Considerations

Normative Ethics: Ethical frameworks consider the role of norms in guiding moral behavior and decision-making.

Norm Violation: Ethical dilemmas arise when personal values conflict with societal norms, requiring individuals to navigate moral and social responsibilities.

Conclusion

Social norms are integral to understanding human behavior and societal dynamics. They provide structure, predictability, and cohesion within communities while influencing individual identity, interpersonal relationships, and cultural practices. Awareness of social norms facilitates effective communication, cooperation, and social integration, promoting harmony and mutual respect in diverse social environments. However, critically evaluating norms allows individuals and societies to adapt, challenge, and evolve toward more inclusive and equitable social norms that reflect changing values and aspirations.

Chapter 49: Definition and Types of Social Norms

Definition: Social norms are unwritten rules or expectations within a society that guide and regulate individuals' behaviors, beliefs, and interactions. They provide a framework for social order and cohesion by defining what is considered acceptable or appropriate in various contexts.

Types of Social Norms:

Descriptive Norms:

Definition: Descriptive norms dictate what behaviors are typically observed or commonly practiced in a specific situation.
Example: Observing others standing in line at a movie theater establishes the norm that queuing is expected behavior.
Injunctive Norms:

Definition: Injunctive norms specify what behaviors are approved or disapproved by others in a society.
Example: Cultural norms that discourage public displays of anger or disrespect reflect injunctive norms about appropriate emotional expression.
How Norms Shape Behavior
Social norms exert significant influence on individual behavior through several mechanisms:

Social Control:

Norms act as a form of social control by regulating behavior and discouraging deviation from accepted standards.

They promote conformity to maintain social order and cohesion.
Normative Influence:

Individuals conform to norms to gain social approval, avoid rejection, or fit in with a group.
Normative influence encourages compliance with social expectations to achieve acceptance and avoid social sanctions.
Internalization:

Over time, individuals internalize societal norms, integrating them into their personal beliefs and values.
Internalized norms guide self-regulation and decision-making, shaping individual identity and behavior.
Changing and Challenging Norms
Social norms are dynamic and subject to change over time due to various factors:

Social Change:

Norms evolve in response to cultural shifts, technological advancements, and generational differences.
Changing societal values and beliefs influence the adaptation or transformation of existing norms.
Deviance and Innovation:

Challenging norms can lead to social innovation and progress by questioning established practices and advocating for alternative behaviors.
Deviance from norms may provoke resistance or social sanctions but can also spur cultural and social change.
Cultural Variability:

Norms vary across cultures and subcultures, reflecting diverse values, traditions, and social expectations.

Cultural diversity contributes to the complexity and adaptation of norms within global and multicultural societies.
Conclusion
Understanding social norms is crucial for comprehending human behavior, societal norms provide structure and predictability in social interactions while influencing individual identity, community dynamics, and cultural practices. Recognizing the influence of norms facilitates effective communication, cooperation, and social integration, fostering mutual understanding and respect within diverse communities.

Chapter 50: Prejudice and Stereotypes

Prejudice and stereotypes are complex social phenomena that profoundly impact individuals, groups, and societies. Understanding their roots, effects, and strategies to combat them is essential for promoting inclusivity and social justice.

The Roots of Prejudice
Definition: Prejudice refers to negative attitudes, beliefs, and feelings toward individuals or groups based on their perceived characteristics, such as race, ethnicity, gender, religion, or socioeconomic status.

Causes and Origins:

Socialization and Cultural Influences:

Prejudice can be learned through socialization processes, where cultural norms, media portrayals, and family beliefs shape attitudes toward different social groups.
Historical and societal narratives often perpetuate biases and stereotypes, influencing intergroup relations.
Cognitive Biases:

Cognitive processes such as categorization and generalization contribute to the formation of stereotypes.
Confirmation bias reinforces existing beliefs by selectively interpreting information that aligns with prejudiced views.
Social Identity Theory:

Prejudice can arise from individuals' need to maintain a positive social identity by denigrating outgroups.
Ingroup favoritism and outgroup derogation serve psychological needs for belonging and self-esteem.
Effects of Stereotyping
Definition: Stereotypes are simplified and generalized beliefs about individuals or groups based on their membership in a particular category.

Impact:

Stereotype Threat:

Individuals may experience stereotype threat, where awareness of negative stereotypes about their group impairs performance and undermines confidence.
This phenomenon can affect academic achievement, job performance, and mental health outcomes.
Social Exclusion and Discrimination:

Stereotypes contribute to social exclusion and discriminatory practices, limiting opportunities and perpetuating inequalities.
Discriminatory behaviors based on stereotypes reinforce social hierarchies and marginalization.
Psychological Effects:

Stereotypes can lead to internalized oppression, where individuals adopt negative stereotypes about their own group.
Psychological distress, low self-esteem, and diminished well-being are common outcomes of experiencing or internalizing stereotypes.
Strategies to Combat Prejudice and Stereotypes
Promoting Social Justice:

Education and Awareness:

Increasing awareness of biases, stereotypes, and their consequences fosters critical thinking and empathy. Education initiatives promote cultural competence and challenge misinformation about marginalized groups.
Intergroup Contact Theory:

Positive interactions between diverse groups reduce prejudice by fostering empathy, understanding, and cooperation. Personal relationships across group boundaries humanize others and challenge stereotypes.
Legislation and Policy:

Legal protections against discrimination and hate crimes mitigate systemic biases and promote equal rights. Policies that support diversity, equity, and inclusion in workplaces and institutions combat institutionalized prejudice.
Media Representation:

Responsible media portrayals that counter stereotypes and showcase diverse perspectives promote social cohesion and tolerance. Media literacy initiatives empower individuals to critically analyze and challenge biased representations.
Conclusion

Prejudice and stereotypes undermine social cohesion and perpetuate inequalities by influencing attitudes, behaviors, and institutional practices. Addressing their roots, effects, and implementing strategies to combat them is crucial for promoting a more equitable and inclusive society. By fostering empathy, challenging biases, and advocating for social justice, individuals and communities can work towards dismantling prejudice and creating environments where diversity is celebrated and respected.

Chapter 51: Identity – The Self in Society

Identity, encompassing both personal and social dimensions, plays a pivotal role in shaping individuals' perceptions, interactions, and experiences within society. Understanding the formation, complexities, and challenges of identity provides insights into how individuals navigate their roles and relationships.

Formation of Social Identity
Definition: Social identity refers to the part of an individual's self-concept that derives from their membership in social groups, such as gender, ethnicity, nationality, religion, or profession.

Key Aspects:

Categorization and Identification:

Individuals categorize themselves and others based on shared characteristics, affiliations, or roles.
Identification with social groups provides a sense of belonging, shared identity, and collective goals.
Social Comparison:

Social identity involves comparing oneself with others within and outside one's group.
Group membership influences perceptions of self-worth, status, and societal roles.
Identity Salience:

The importance of different social identities varies across contexts and influences behavior and self-presentation.
Situational cues and social contexts may activate specific identities, shaping attitudes and behaviors.
Intersectionality and Multiple Identities
Definition: Intersectionality examines how multiple social identities (e.g., race, gender, class) intersect to shape unique experiences of privilege, discrimination, and social power.

Key Concepts:

Complexity of Identity:

Intersectionality acknowledges that individuals embody multiple identities simultaneously, influencing their perspectives and experiences.
Intersecting identities interact in complex ways, shaping access to resources, opportunities, and social recognition.
Social Hierarchies:

Intersectional analysis highlights how systems of power and oppression (e.g., racism, sexism) intersect to create unique social positions.

Marginalized individuals may experience compounded discrimination or invisibility due to intersecting identities.
Advocacy and Social Change:

Intersectionality informs advocacy efforts by recognizing the diversity of experiences within marginalized communities. Promoting inclusive policies and practices acknowledges intersectional identities and addresses systemic inequalities.
Identity Crisis and Resolution
Definition: Identity crisis refers to a period of uncertainty and exploration in which individuals question their values, beliefs, and identity choices. Resolution involves integrating diverse aspects of the self into a cohesive identity.

Developmental Processes:

Adolescent Identity Formation:

Adolescents explore various roles, beliefs, and relationships to establish a sense of identity.
Peer influence, family dynamics, and cultural contexts shape identity development during adolescence.
Adult Identity Development:

Identity continues to evolve across the lifespan through personal experiences, life transitions, and evolving social roles.
Resolving identity crises involves introspection, self-discovery, and integration of personal and social identities.
Cultural and Contextual Influences:

Cultural norms, societal expectations, and historical events influence individual identity formation and resolution.
Cultural identity affirmation and pride contribute to psychological well-being and community resilience.
Conclusion

Identity encompasses the complex interplay of personal experiences, social contexts, and cultural affiliations that shape individuals' sense of self and belonging. Understanding the formation of social identity, intersectionality, and the dynamics of identity crisis and resolution enhances empathy, promotes inclusivity, and informs strategies for fostering personal growth and social justice. Embracing diverse identities and recognizing their intersectional nature enriches societal discourse and strengthens community bonds based on mutual respect and understanding.

Chapter 52: Social Perception – Understanding Others

Social perception involves the cognitive processes through which individuals interpret and understand the behavior, intentions, and traits of others within social contexts. It plays a crucial role in forming impressions, making decisions, and navigating interpersonal relationships.

Processes of Social Perception
Definition: Processes of social perception refer to the mental operations used to gather, interpret, and integrate information about others.

Key Aspects:

Perceiving and Encoding Social Information:

Individuals observe and selectively attend to relevant cues from others' verbal and nonverbal behaviors.
Encoding involves translating sensory information into meaningful representations, influenced by attention and cognitive schemas.
Forming Impressions:

Initial impressions are formed rapidly based on limited information, often guided by stereotypes, personal experiences, and contextual cues.
Impressions may be influenced by attractiveness, similarity, perceived competence, and warmth.
Attribution Processes:

Attribution involves explaining the causes of behavior, either attributing it to internal factors (dispositional attribution) or external factors (situational attribution).
Attribution biases, such as fundamental attribution error and actor-observer bias, shape interpretations of others' actions.
Errors in Social Perception
Definition: Errors in social perception refer to cognitive biases and perceptual distortions that lead to inaccurate interpretations of others' behavior or characteristics.

Common Biases:

Fundamental Attribution Error:

Tendency to attribute others' behaviors to internal traits while underestimating situational influences.
Leads to overestimating dispositional factors and underestimating external factors in explaining behavior.
Stereotyping and Prejudice:

Stereotypes are oversimplified beliefs about social groups, influencing perceptions and expectations.

Prejudice involves negative attitudes and emotions toward individuals based on group membership, distorting social perceptions.
Confirmation Bias:

Preference for information that confirms existing beliefs or stereotypes, leading to selective attention and interpretation of social cues.
Reinforces initial impressions and maintains cognitive schemas.
Improving Social Perceptiveness
Enhancing Accuracy and Empathy:

Active Listening and Empathic Understanding:

Active listening involves attentive engagement and validation of others' perspectives and emotions.
Empathy promotes perspective-taking and emotional resonance, fostering understanding and rapport.
Cognitive Flexibility:

Adopting a flexible mindset allows for considering alternative explanations and challenging initial impressions.
Open-mindedness reduces reliance on stereotypes and biases in social judgments.
Awareness of Bias and Self-Reflection:

Recognizing personal biases and cognitive shortcuts encourages critical reflection on social perceptions.
Mindfulness of situational influences promotes more accurate attributions and interpretations of behavior.
Conclusion

Social perception is a dynamic process influenced by cognitive, emotional, and social factors that shape how individuals understand and interact with others. By understanding the processes of social perception, recognizing common errors and biases, and actively cultivating social perceptiveness, individuals can enhance interpersonal relationships, promote empathy, and navigate social complexities with greater accuracy and insight. Developing a nuanced understanding of social perception contributes to more effective communication, conflict resolution, and ethical decision-making in diverse social contexts.

Chapter 53: The Importance of Social Support

Social support encompasses various forms of assistance, empathy, and encouragement exchanged between individuals within social networks. It plays a critical role in promoting psychological well-being, resilience, and overall quality of life.

Types of Social Support
1. Emotional Support:

Definition: Emotional support involves empathy, encouragement, and reassurance provided by others during times of stress, sadness, or uncertainty.
Role: It helps individuals feel understood, validated, and cared for, enhancing emotional resilience and coping mechanisms.
2. Instrumental Support:

Definition: Instrumental support includes tangible aid such as financial assistance, practical help with tasks, or logistical support.
Role: It addresses practical needs and challenges, reducing stress and enhancing problem-solving capabilities.
3. Informational Support:

Definition: Informational support includes guidance, advice, and information provided to help individuals make informed decisions or understand challenging situations.
Role: It promotes effective decision-making, enhances problem-solving skills, and reduces uncertainty.
4. Appraisal Support:

Definition: Appraisal support involves constructive feedback, affirmation, and evaluation of one's thoughts, feelings, or behaviors.
Role: It helps individuals gain clarity, perspective, and self-awareness, fostering personal growth and adaptive coping strategies.
Benefits of Social Support Networks
1. Psychological Well-being:

Role: Social support networks provide a sense of belonging, security, and acceptance, reducing feelings of loneliness and isolation.
Impact: They contribute to improved mental health outcomes, including reduced anxiety, depression, and stress.

2. Physical Health:

Role: Strong social connections and support networks are associated with better physical health outcomes.
Impact: They promote immune function, cardiovascular health, and faster recovery from illness or injury.
3. Coping with Stress:

Role: Social support buffers the impact of stressful life events and adversity.
Impact: It enhances resilience, adaptive coping strategies, and the ability to manage and overcome challenges.
4. Enhanced Quality of Life:

Role: Supportive relationships foster a sense of fulfillment, happiness, and life satisfaction.
Impact: They promote positive life experiences, meaningful connections, and a sense of purpose.
Building and Maintaining Supportive Relationships
1. Reciprocity and Trust:

Building: Establish mutual trust, reciprocity, and reliability in relationships.
Maintaining: Demonstrate consistency, responsiveness, and genuine concern for others' well-being.
2. Effective Communication:

Building: Foster open communication, active listening, and empathy in interactions.
Maintaining: Address misunderstandings promptly, express appreciation, and resolve conflicts constructively.
3. Nurturing Connections:

Building: Cultivate shared interests, experiences, and activities that strengthen bonds.

Maintaining: Prioritize quality time, celebrate milestones, and offer support during challenging times.

4. Seeking and Offering Support:

Building: Be proactive in offering support and seeking assistance when needed.

Maintaining: Balance giving and receiving support to sustain reciprocal relationships and mutual benefit.

Conclusion

Social support networks are fundamental to individuals' well-being, resilience, and ability to navigate life's challenges effectively. By understanding the types and benefits of social support, as well as strategies for building and maintaining supportive relationships, individuals can cultivate meaningful connections, enhance their coping mechanisms, and promote overall health and happiness. Investing in social support fosters a sense of community, belonging, and mutual empowerment, enriching both personal and collective experiences in diverse social contexts.

Chapter 54: Essential Social Skills for Success

1. Communication Skills:

Definition: Effective verbal and nonverbal communication is essential for expressing thoughts clearly, listening actively, and understanding others' perspectives.

Role: It fosters mutual understanding, reduces misunderstandings, and enhances relationship building.

2. Empathy and Emotional Intelligence:

Definition: Empathy involves understanding and sharing others' emotions, while emotional intelligence encompasses awareness, regulation, and utilization of emotions in social interactions.

Role: They promote empathy, enhance emotional regulation, and facilitate supportive relationships.

3. Assertiveness:

Definition: Assertiveness involves expressing one's needs, beliefs, and opinions confidently and respectfully while considering others' perspectives.

Role: It fosters self-confidence, improves conflict resolution skills, and promotes healthy boundaries.

4. Interpersonal Skills:

Definition: Interpersonal skills encompass building rapport, showing respect, and fostering positive relationships through effective communication and mutual respect.

Role: They enhance collaboration, teamwork, and cooperation in diverse social and professional settings.

Training and Enhancing Social Skills

1. Social Skills Training Programs:

Purpose: Structured programs provide education and practice opportunities to develop specific social skills, such as assertiveness, active listening, and conflict resolution.

Role: They improve social competence, self-confidence, and adaptability in various social contexts.

2. Role-Playing and Simulation Exercises:

Purpose: Role-playing activities simulate real-life scenarios to practice social skills, decision-making, and problem-solving under different circumstances.

Role: They enhance communication effectiveness, empathy, and adaptive behavior in challenging situations.

3. Feedback and Reflection:

Purpose: Soliciting feedback and reflecting on social interactions facilitate self-awareness, identify strengths and areas for improvement, and refine social skills.
Role: They promote continuous learning, personal growth, and refinement of interpersonal effectiveness.
Social Skills in Different Contexts
1. Personal Relationships:

Role: Effective social skills nurture intimate connections, strengthen emotional bonds, and promote mutual support and understanding.
Impact: They enhance relationship satisfaction, communication openness, and conflict resolution abilities.
2. Professional Settings:

Role: Social skills are critical for networking, collaboration, leadership, and career advancement in the workplace.
Impact: They foster professional relationships, teamwork, and productivity, contributing to organizational success and professional growth.
3. Cultural Competence:

Role: Cultural sensitivity and awareness of social norms and customs facilitate respectful and inclusive interactions in diverse cultural settings.
Impact: They promote cross-cultural understanding, reduce misunderstandings, and build trust and cooperation across cultural boundaries.
Conclusion

Developing and enhancing social skills is an ongoing process that contributes to personal growth, meaningful relationships, and professional success. By cultivating essential social skills, participating in structured training programs, and adapting social behaviors to diverse contexts, individuals can navigate social interactions with confidence, empathy, and effectiveness. Investing in social skill development fosters resilience, enhances interpersonal connections, and supports personal and professional achievements in a dynamic and interconnected world.

Chapter 55: The Process of Socialization

Socialization is the lifelong process through which individuals acquire the knowledge, values, norms, and behaviors that enable them to function effectively within their society. It begins from infancy and continues throughout one's life, shaping how individuals perceive themselves and interact with others.

Agents of Socialization
1. Family:

Role: Families are the primary agents of socialization during early childhood, transmitting cultural norms, values, and behaviors to children through direct instruction, modeling, and reinforcement.
Impact: Family socialization influences foundational beliefs, attitudes, and interpersonal skills that individuals carry into adulthood.
2. Peers:

Role: Peers become increasingly influential during adolescence and beyond, providing opportunities for social interaction, learning social roles, and experimenting with identity and behavior.
Impact: Peer socialization fosters social skills, establishes norms of conduct, and shapes individuals' attitudes and behaviors within their peer groups.
3. School and Education:

Role: Educational institutions reinforce societal norms, values, and knowledge through formal curriculum, extracurricular activities, and interactions with peers and teachers.
Impact: School socialization promotes academic achievement, social integration, and prepares individuals for roles in society and the workforce.
4. Media and Technology:

Role: Mass media, including television, internet, and social media platforms, shapes attitudes, values, and behaviors by portraying societal norms, influencing cultural trends, and providing information.
Impact: Media socialization contributes to cultural identity formation, consumer behavior, and perceptions of social reality.
Lifelong Socialization
Socialization is an ongoing process that continues throughout adulthood:

Adulthood: Individuals continue to refine their social roles, adapt to changing societal expectations, and acquire new knowledge and skills through work, relationships, and life experiences.
Older Adults: Socialization remains important in later life as individuals adjust to retirement, maintain social networks, and contribute to intergenerational relationships.
Impact of Socialization on Behavior
Socialization influences behavior in several key ways:

Normative Behavior: Individuals conform to societal norms, internalizing expectations for appropriate conduct, values, and beliefs.
Social Roles: Socialization assigns roles and responsibilities within society, shaping occupational choices, family roles, and community participation.

Cultural Adaptation: Socialization facilitates adaptation to cultural practices, customs, and traditions, promoting cultural competence and effective intercultural communication.

Behavioral Patterns: Socialization contributes to the development of behavioral patterns, such as altruism, cooperation, competition, and conformity, that define social interactions and relationships.

Conclusion

The process of socialization is essential for individuals to acquire the skills, knowledge, and behaviors necessary for effective participation in society. By interacting with family, peers, educational institutions, media, and other socializing agents throughout their lives, individuals develop a sense of identity, cultural belonging, and social competence. Understanding the dynamics of socialization underscores its profound impact on behavior, interpersonal relationships, and societal cohesion, highlighting its role in shaping individuals' experiences and contributions within diverse social contexts.

Conclusion: The Interconnectedness of Social Psychological Concepts

Throughout this exploration of social psychology, we have delved into the intricate web of human behavior, relationships, and societal dynamics. The field of social psychology offers profound insights into how individuals perceive themselves and others, navigate social interactions, and contribute to the fabric of society. As we conclude this journey, several key themes emerge that highlight the interconnected nature of social psychological concepts.

Recap of Key Themes
1. Human Connection and Social Interactions:

Social interactions form the foundation of human existence, shaping our identities, beliefs, and behaviors. Whether through familial ties, romantic relationships, or friendships, these interactions influence our emotional well-being and sense of belonging.
2. Psychological Processes and Behavior:

Psychological theories and models provide frameworks for understanding behavior. From cognitive processes and emotional regulation to social perception and decision-making, these processes intricately influence how individuals interpret and respond to their social environment.
3. Influence of Social Norms and Group Dynamics:

Social norms dictate acceptable behavior within a society or group, exerting significant influence on individual actions and decisions. Group dynamics further amplify these norms, shaping group cohesion, leadership dynamics, and collective behaviors.

4. Identity Formation and Socialization:

Identity is shaped through socialization processes that begin in childhood and evolve throughout life. Social identity, influenced by cultural norms and personal experiences, plays a pivotal role in shaping individual beliefs, values, and interactions with others.

5. Impact of Social Support and Communication:

Social support networks provide emotional, informational, and instrumental assistance that enhances resilience and well-being. Effective communication skills facilitate interpersonal connections, conflict resolution, and the exchange of ideas within diverse social contexts.

The Holistic Understanding of Human Connection

By integrating these themes, social psychology offers a holistic understanding of human connection and behavior. It underscores the reciprocal relationship between individuals and their social environment, emphasizing the dynamic interplay between internal psychological processes and external social influences.

Future Directions in Social Psychology Research

As we look to the future, ongoing research in social psychology continues to explore emerging trends and societal shifts. Areas such as digital communication, globalization, cultural diversity, and the impact of technology on social interactions present new avenues for investigation. Understanding these dynamics will further enrich our understanding of human behavior and inform interventions aimed at promoting positive social change.

Final Thoughts
In closing, the study of social psychology is not merely an academic pursuit but a profound exploration of what it means to be human in a social world. It challenges us to critically examine our assumptions, empathize with diverse perspectives, and foster inclusive communities. By embracing the interconnectedness of social psychological concepts, we empower ourselves to navigate complexities, foster meaningful relationships, and contribute positively to society.

Through this journey, may we continue to explore, learn, and apply the principles of social psychology to promote understanding, empathy, and collective well-being in our interconnected world.

Recap of Key Themes in Social Psychology

Human Connection and Social Interactions:

Social interactions are fundamental to human existence, influencing our emotions, behaviors, and relationships. Whether in familial, romantic, or platonic contexts, these interactions shape our identities and contribute to our sense of belonging.
Psychological Processes and Behavior:

Social psychology examines various psychological processes that influence behavior. These include cognitive processes like perception, memory, and decision-making, as well as emotional processes such as regulation and expression. Understanding these processes helps explain how individuals navigate social situations and relationships.
Influence of Social Norms and Group Dynamics:

Social norms are unwritten rules that guide behavior within a society or group. They define what is considered appropriate or acceptable behavior and play a crucial role in social cohesion and conformity. Group dynamics further amplify these norms, affecting leadership dynamics, decision-making processes, and collective behavior.

Identity Formation and Socialization:

Identity formation is influenced by socialization processes that begin in childhood and continue throughout life. Social identity, shaped by cultural norms, values, and experiences, affects how individuals perceive themselves and others. It plays a significant role in shaping beliefs, values, and behaviors within societal and cultural contexts.

Impact of Social Support and Communication:

Social support networks provide emotional, informational, and instrumental assistance that enhances well-being and resilience. Effective communication skills are essential for building and maintaining relationships, resolving conflicts, and fostering understanding across diverse social contexts.

Conclusion

These key themes underscore the complexity and interconnectedness of social psychological concepts. By examining how individuals perceive themselves and others, navigate social norms, form identities, and communicate within groups, social psychology offers valuable insights into human behavior and societal dynamics. Understanding these themes fosters empathy, promotes positive social interactions, and informs interventions aimed at improving individual and collective well-being.

Continued research and exploration in social psychology are crucial for addressing contemporary challenges, promoting inclusivity, and enhancing our understanding of human nature in an ever-evolving social landscape.

The Holistic Understanding of Human Connection

The holistic understanding of human connection in social psychology encompasses a comprehensive view of how individuals interact, form relationships, and influence one another within social contexts. This concept underscores several key aspects:

Interpersonal Relationships: Social psychology examines the dynamics of interpersonal relationships, including familial, romantic, and platonic connections. It explores how individuals perceive and interpret social cues, communicate emotions, and navigate conflicts within these relationships.

Social Influence: Human connection involves the mutual influence individuals exert on each other's thoughts, feelings, and behaviors. Social psychology studies how group norms, peer pressure, and cultural values shape individual actions and decisions, highlighting the interplay between conformity and autonomy.

Emotional Bonds: Understanding human connection involves exploring the emotional bonds that individuals form with others. This includes empathy, compassion, and emotional support networks that contribute to psychological well-being and resilience in the face of challenges.

Identity and Belonging: Social psychology investigates how social identities (e.g., cultural, ethnic, gender) influence individuals' sense of belonging and self-concept. It explores the impact of societal expectations, stereotypes, and prejudice on identity formation and social integration.

Communication and Interaction: Effective communication skills are pivotal in establishing and maintaining human connections. Social psychology examines verbal and nonverbal communication patterns, interpersonal skills, and the role of active listening in fostering meaningful relationships.

Cultural and Contextual Factors: Human connection is shaped by cultural norms, societal structures, and historical contexts. Social psychology acknowledges the diversity of human experiences and perspectives, emphasizing the importance of cultural competence and understanding in promoting mutual respect and collaboration.

Implications and Applications

By comprehensively understanding human connection, social psychology informs strategies for promoting positive social interactions, conflict resolution, and community building. It underscores the significance of empathy, respect for diversity, and ethical considerations in fostering inclusive environments where individuals thrive emotionally and socially.

Future Directions
Continued research in social psychology will further illuminate the complexities of human connection in a rapidly changing world. Emerging topics such as digital communication, globalization, and the influence of technology on social dynamics offer new avenues for exploration. By integrating interdisciplinary perspectives and advancing theoretical frameworks, social psychology continues to contribute to our understanding of human behavior and the promotion of healthy, supportive communities.

Future Directions in Social Psychology Research

Future directions in social psychology research are shaped by emerging trends, technological advancements, and evolving societal challenges. Here are some key areas of focus:

Digital and Virtual Interactions: As digital communication platforms continue to evolve, there is a growing interest in understanding how online interactions influence social behaviors, identities, and relationships. Research may explore topics such as social media use, virtual communities, online identity construction, and the impact of digital communication on mental health and well-being.

Cultural and Global Perspectives: Social psychology increasingly emphasizes the need for cross-cultural research to explore how cultural norms, values, and beliefs shape social interactions and behaviors. Comparative studies can deepen our understanding of universal psychological processes while highlighting cultural variations in social cognition, emotion regulation, and interpersonal relationships.

Social Justice and Inequality: Addressing issues of social justice, equity, and inequality remains a critical area of research. Social psychologists examine the psychological mechanisms underlying prejudice, discrimination, and intergroup relations, as well as strategies for promoting social justice, reducing bias, and fostering inclusive societies.

Environmental and Pro-Social Behavior: With growing concerns about environmental sustainability and collective action, social psychology explores how individuals perceive and respond to environmental issues. Research may focus on pro-environmental behavior, sustainable lifestyles, and the role of social norms, collective efficacy, and behavioral interventions in promoting environmental conservation.

Health and Well-being: Social psychology contributes to understanding the psychosocial factors influencing health behaviors, health disparities, and healthcare utilization. Future research may explore the impact of social support networks, stigma reduction strategies, and behavioral interventions on promoting mental health, resilience, and overall well-being.

Technology and Human Interaction: Advances in technology, such as artificial intelligence and virtual reality, offer new opportunities to study human-computer interactions and their implications for social behavior. Research may investigate topics such as digital empathy, virtual social presence, and the ethical implications of technological innovations on interpersonal relationships and social norms.

Intersectionality and Multiple Identities: Recognizing the complexity of human identity, social psychology increasingly explores how intersecting social categories (e.g., race, gender, sexuality, socioeconomic status) shape individuals' experiences of identity, privilege, and discrimination. Intersectional approaches highlight the need for nuanced understandings of social identity dynamics and their implications for social policy and practice.

Behavioral Change and Intervention Strategies: Social psychology contributes to developing effective interventions aimed at promoting positive behavioral change, from health promotion to conflict resolution and social activism. Future research may focus on identifying motivational factors, designing persuasive communication strategies, and evaluating the long-term impact of behavioral interventions in diverse contexts.

Conclusion

The future of social psychology research is dynamic and multifaceted, driven by ongoing societal transformations and interdisciplinary collaborations. By addressing complex social issues, integrating diverse perspectives, and leveraging innovative methodologies, social psychologists contribute to advancing knowledge, fostering social change, and promoting well-being in an interconnected world.